LET THEM HEAR

AN EAR SURGEON'S
JOYFUL EXPERIENCE WITH
ENABLING PEOPLE TO HEAR

JOSEPH B. ROBERSON, JR., M.D.

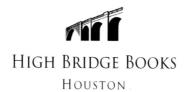

HIGH BRIDGE BOOKS
HOUSTON

Let Them Hear
by Joseph B. Roberson, Jr., M.D.

Printed in the United States of America
ISBN (Paperback): 978-1-946615-33-6
ISBN (eBook): 978-1-946615-34-3

High Bridge Books titles may be purchased in bulk for educational, business, fundraising, or sales promotional use. For information, please contact High Bridge Books via www.HighBridgeBooks.com/contact.

Published in Houston, Texas by High Bridge Books

My Heavenly Father

I relish the thought of the time when I meet you face to face to thank You for the joy and privilege You grant me to work as a surgeon during my life on this planet. I have learned You are generous, unchangingly dedicated in love toward man, gloriously magnificent, and filled with sacrifice and resolute effort toward relationship. You have given me incredible access to watch You work—even allowing me to be an integral part in many situations. My joy expresses itself in hoping to please You consistent with Colossians 3:23-24. I have already been given a strong reward.

Earthly Fathers (and Mothers, too)

One thing on earth simply slays me—it enlarges and touches my heart within moments—to see a loving father yearning to care for his child in need with his strength and sacrifice. Nothing stirs me more to go to war on your behalf and on behalf of your child—enduring any hardship to produce the best I can possibly achieve. May your efforts for your children bring blessings beyond what you hope.

Contents

Acknowledgments

SURGERY IS A LONG ROAD—11 years of training beyond college, with no salary for the first four years and a salary less than $20,000 per year for the next seven, while raising three children just to get there. The demands, post-training, have been at least as large as well in different ways.

Through the entire process, one person—my wife Julia—has been my greatest stalwart and support. She has steadily maintained a warm and fruitful home during very demanding times while remaining dedicated to a calling of her own for many years. She loves me and cheers me on to greater things, keeping her feet in this world but her eyes on the next. To allow me and encourage me to add the requirements of a Foundation to my challenging life is above and beyond—just as she has blessed me in our 35 years of marriage. Thank you doesn't come close, my dearest. You are the most precious thing to me on this earth.

My children Caitlin, Baxter, and Haley—your participation in most all the international events in this book took courage, intrepidness, and inspiration. I have been so proud of you putting your hearts out there as we have experienced these events together. Hearing and watching your reactions have brought home the greatest things I have learned about life, the world, and the Maker of this world. I am privileged to be your dad.

The Let Them Hear Foundation would never have occurred without two things: friends who both encouraged me and participated on the Board of LTHF—Dale, Margaret, Kirk, Jim, Nersi, Bob, Les, Frank, and their significant others in some cases—as well as the patients and friends who have donated to make these trips possible. While I can't let you do the surgery, your presence to share in the miracles of hearing is one of the greatest joys of my life. I trust you grasp what a difference you have made in the lives of children.

The staff of The Let Them Hear Foundation have worked tirelessly over the years, inspiring and being inspired, leading and being led, blessing and being blessed. Paul, Rob, Sheri, Tracy, and dozens of others, you have made miracles happen. I am honored to have worked beside you.

Introduction

I AM AN EAR SURGEON and, as I have come to realize over the course of my career, was created to be one. Through the surgeries I have performed, I have helped over 5,000 people hear clearly with a variety of surgical procedures—some hearing for the very first time. The joy of witnessing patients listen to their loved ones' voices for the first time has been unspeakable.

As I watch people early in their lives—including my children in their 20s and their friends—strive to figure out their life work, it challenges me to examine my own work choices. If you are considering your life's work as you read this book, try to answer one of the greatest questions in life which is not just what you are here for but who you are here for.

Although some of these ear surgeries were performed for patients at my clinic in Silicon Valley at the California Ear Institute, I have performed many through the Let Them Hear Foundation (LTHF) for children in third-world countries such as Myanmar, a place where few can afford or provide such procedures at regular cost.

Since most of the stories in this book happened thanks to the Foundation, allow me a few lines to share the organization's mission and how it works.

Let Them Hear Foundation is a 501c(3) non-profit organization my wife Julia and I founded in 2002. Its purpose is to spread the complex hearing technology we have been blessed with in the United States to people in foreign nations and to provide cochlear implants—a surgery that helps enable deaf patients to hear (I'll explain more later).

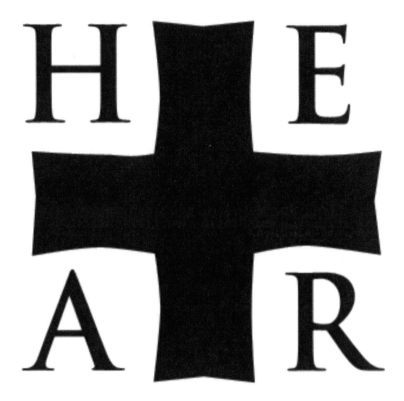

Starting cochlear implant programs around the world has become our mission. It takes time and significant resources, but we work in-country to foster these programs so local surgeons and physicians can continue providing cochlear implants long after we have left. It's a manifestation of the well-known "teach a man to fish" doctrine.

So far, we have initiated 11 different cochlear implants centers in countries around the globe. A few include Costa Rica, Peru, Singapore, Indonesia, Nepal, China (we have put several there), and Bulgaria.

We have also been able to bring aid to folks here in the states through the Foundation. Previously, most insurance companies didn't cover single ear cochlear implants, and no insurance companies covered bilateral cochlear implants (yes, two are definitely better than one, as you might expect)–a rather expensive procedure, priced at a hefty $50,000-$55,000 per ear. It took patients who paid for their own procedure years to pay it off. Worse yet, some patients went without.

However, after wrangling a legal team of attorneys from across the nation together, we had them take cases for cochlear implant patients to make the procedure more readily available. Case by case (1054 of them), filing both individual and class action lawsuits against specific insurance companies who refused to cover the procedure, this legal advocacy team established cochlear implants as a means of treatment for severe to profound sensorineural hearing loss.

Today, this team of incredible attorneys led by Sheri Byrne-Haber JD of LTHF single-handedly won this battle. We have since shut the program down. The legal team obviously worked itself out of need, which is a good thing.

As stated earlier, we also implement programs in nations where most citizens are too poor for a cochlear implantation. But before any training center is set up, we have to travel in person to these countries and teach this delicate surgical procedure, which can be exciting and harrowing–sometimes both.

A typical LTHF trip lasts anywhere from a week to 10 days. The size of our group varies–usually anywhere from 10 to 40 people. A day or two after we land, our team meets the families of the patients, discusses aspects of the surgery with them–pre-surgery prep, recovery times, how to ready their patient (usually a child), etc.– and how to take care of their patient after the surgery. We also go over the financial commitment we expect from them, which can range from \$100-\$500 depending on their need. The cost to us is many times this amount, and this small amount of assistance is not material in the overall budget. It's not to turn a profit but, rather, gives the families a chance to receive the surgery as a service rather than charity; it honors them.

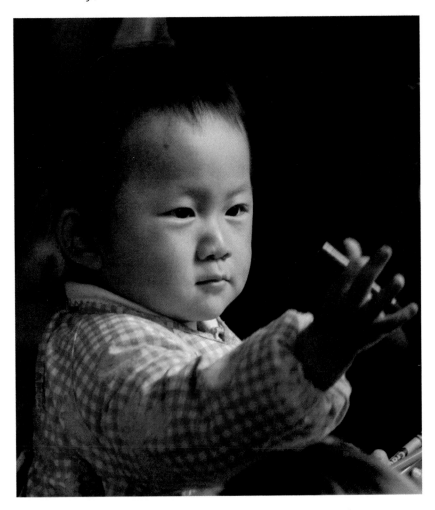

Deaf three-year-old girl from China
who received an LTHF cochlear implant

A couple of days later, we're performing the actual surgeries. Each takes roughly an hour and a half, and, as is the case for outpatients in the United States, we keep the children overnight to make sure there aren't any complications resulting from the surgery. A few days later, they're back in the clinic or hospital where we have set up shop. That's when we test the cochlear implants (which look like hearing aids) we inserted via surgery. That's when the truly incredible moment—in which they hear sound for the first time—occurs.

The trip is a week of condensed intensity, one we'd never take people unexperienced in medicine on, but that moment at the very end of it makes it all—the challenges, difficulties, hardships, and discomforts—worth it.

As of now, we're proceeding with and planning more trips. We're also praying over our plans for LTHF's next few years and where to allocate funding a former patient posthumously donated. When you think of us, please feel free to join in this prayer.

In the grand scheme of things, deafness, or hearing loss, is one of the most common birth defects; many people don't know that. In fact, if every child that will be born deaf or with impaired hearing in the next 10 years held hands, they would make a human chain long enough to stretch around the earth two-and-a-half times. The disability is crippling in that it severely affects an individual's quality of life and, if it isn't treated early in life, severely hampers their ability to learn vital communication skills with severe impact on job opportunities.

The Lord said in Matthew 26:11, "For you always have the poor with you," and it's my heart to help people who can't afford the care they need. However, as a steward of medical skills, I want to leverage both my resources and abilities, so others can help those in need, to offer the greatest amount of aid possible and empower others to do so as well. In this model, we also get the most of the precious funds others entrust to us—in effect promoting as high a philanthropic return on investment that we can achieve by leaving professionals in place to continue this work.

I can't express how blessed I feel to work in this field at this time in history. Our resources here in the states (particularly in California's Silicon Valley, the greatest wealth-producing region in the history of the world) are abundant—therefore I feel led to share the knowledge, technology, equipment, and God's other many blessings with the world around us—to serve as His outstretched arms. Our greatest privilege comes when someone asks us, "Why do you do this?" and we get to explain.

I realize you may not share my desire to follow Jesus, but I include my heart in many of these stories because that is a part of me. You need to know that to understand my experience. I am sure you'll allow me that privilege just like I respect your right to make your own decision regarding the One I have come to love and value immensely.

Throughout this book, I'll take you into operating and recovery rooms, hospitals, and clinics, in both the United States and countries overseas. Many of these stories have to do with bringing hearing to patients' lives, while some are from experiences during broader surgical training. It's my hope that through these stories, I won't only convey experiences and the joy of my work but perhaps help you find a deeper joy in the vocation and calling you find yourself in right now. If you are young and feel called to medicine, read these stories and realize the phenomenal blessing, responsibility, and effort it takes from you and those you love to do this right. Plus, these stories are simply too good not to share!

1

A New Sense

IMAGINE YOU'RE INSIDE a hospital room. Nurses and doctors bustle, moving equipment, speaking in rushed phrases, acronymically, reading complex information on blinking monitors that hum with electricity. A baby has just been born. Father and mother both catch a moment of respite as the extended family waits eagerly outside. It's a picturesque moment and, though somewhat typical, miraculous; life has been created and brought forth into the world.

The baby is washed, weighed, and wrapped in a blanket, equally pink and blue. The child has been crying and continues crying even after being handed to its mother. She whispers comforting words to soothe the child, but the crying only continues.

Deafness ... It's not a virus or disease or something you can see. Rather, it's usually hereditary when present at birth, caused by certain genetic issues. Some children are born deaf—about one out of every 1,000—while others are born with partial deafness and lose it gradually. In some cases, patients come down with meningitis or other diseases, which, in turn, deteriorates their hearing.

In the fictional scenario above, neither of the parents suffer from deafness. They both have excellent hearing. But unbeknownst to them, their new child will suffer from an ailment neither of them—nor the doctors and nurses present—could have foreseen or predicted.

Ninety-five percent of children born with deafness are born to parents with perfectly good hearing. Nothing in these children's appearance alludes to their disability. Even their ears are, on the outside, totally normal. However, down deep in the inner ear lies the cochlea—a small, seashell-shaped organ buried deep within the inner ear, made no less important by its size (or lack thereof).

As a physician, I specialize in cochlear implants. It's difficult to convey the feeling of helping another human hear, but before I attempt any articulation, it's appropriate to explain the cochlea's function.

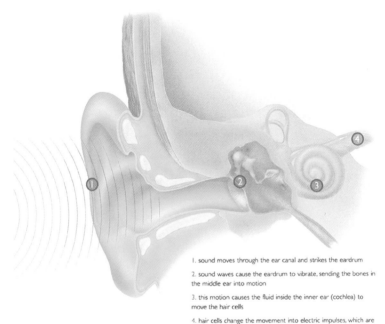

1. sound moves through the ear canal and strikes the eardrum

2. sound waves cause the eardrum to vibrate, sending the bones in the middle ear into motion

3. this motion causes the fluid inside the inner ear (cochlea) to move the hair cells

4. hair cells change the movement into electric impulses, which are sent to the hearing nerve into the brain; you hear sound

When the ear picks up a sound, it sends it down the ear canal and to the eardrum as a series of vibrations. The vibrations pass through the amplification system of the middle ear and then enter the fluid in the inner ear. The vibrations stimulate the cochlea's nerve cells—just as water would move and shift grass submersed in a river bed—any vibrations coming through the fluid have the same effect a boat would have passing over the grass.

Small, "hair cells" (they aren't actually hair, that's simply what they're called) pick up the vibrations fire nerve signals, sending electric impulses to the brain via what physicians call the "eighth cranial nerve," the final bridge in a sound's journey to the brain. The transmission is translated by the brain as a sound over 10,000 nerve fibers arising in the cochlea.

Despite the cochlea's small size, its importance in this seemingly mechanical process can't be understated. Without it, all other parts of the ear and their functions are rendered utterly useless.

The vast majority of deaf patients have cochleae that lack these vital hair cells, resulting in deafness. In short, their ears can pick up sound but have no way of transducing into signals for the brain.

If it isn't treated quickly, deafness can have devastating effects on a child's ability to communicate, since a child learning to speak must be able to hear themselves. The issue becomes exacerbated by the science of development—their first five years of life are the most critical for speech development, and a vast majority of that occurs before they even turn three. If they miss this window of time, it's far more difficult for them to learn to speak later in life—in fact, it can be impossible. In short, an early intervention not only gives them hearing but the chance to learn to speak unhindered. Therefore, the earlier I can operate on a patient, the better. Although a one-year-old is typically the youngest who should be operated on, I have done an implant on children as young as four months old. If this critical period of development is missed, it can never be regained.

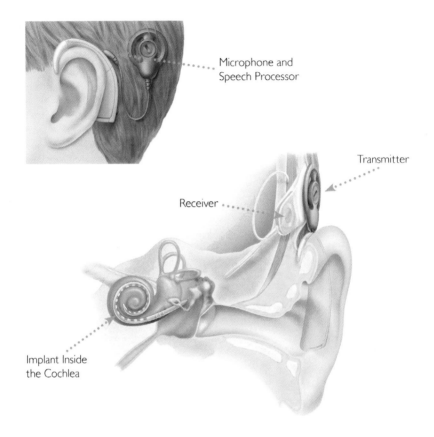

Microphone and
Speech Processor

Transmitter

Receiver

Implant Inside
the Cochlea

The procedure is a delicate one—and that's putting it mildly. The surgical process begins when we drill a small recess in the bone of a patient's skull to hold the main portion of the implant under the skin. The implant comes attached to a delicate wire on which are electrodes. We then make an opening no larger than a millimeter in the cochlea and pass the electrode implant into it. The implant works by receiving sound through a microphone outside the skin, sending it to the body of the implant where a sophisticated computer processes the sound, sending it to the electrodes in the cochlea.

Each electrode bypasses the missing hair cells and stimulates the eighth cranial nerve directly, which takes the electrical signal to the brain and produces sound. It's programmed to deliver frequency to the proper places along the interior of the cochlea, firing thousands of times in a minute. In a sense, it tunes the cochlea.

We started using these sorts of implants in the 1980s. They were crude and couldn't come close to the effectiveness of their modern counterpart, but we were ecstatic when they helped our patients hear anything. The technology has progressed incredibly rapidly over the last 20 or 25 years so that patients can now experience sound that's much closer to what those without deafness hear.

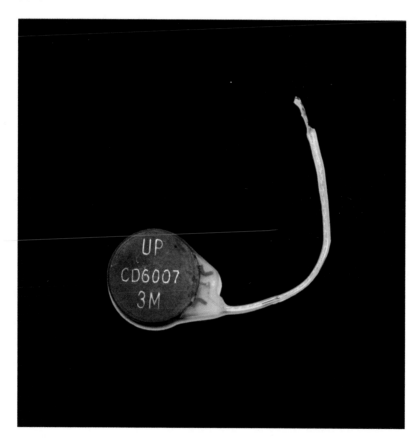

One of the first cochlear implants circa 1988.
Note the single implanted electrode.

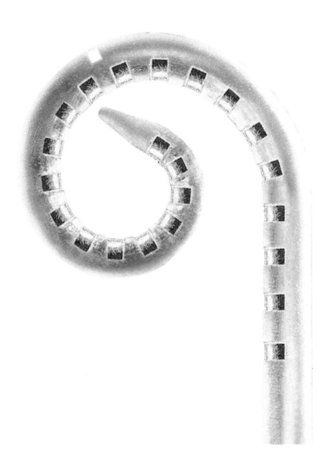

*Modern cochlear implants have multiple electrodes
and produce much better sound*

After waking from surgery, patients and their parents are allowed to recover before they come to my office to have the implant turned on and tuned. Electrode by electrode, we test the frequency of the implant using a combination of magnets and radio coils; one set is inside the implant and the other, a matching external counterpart.

Using the external components, the electrical current is amplified, and the sound coming from the implant grows louder and louder until the patient can perceive any noise.

As unscientific and rudimentary as it seems, a conversation over the phone is one of the best gauges for measuring a patient's hearing level after an implant. Such an exchange removes all elements of non-verbal communication—facial expression, hand motions, body positioning, etc.—and isolates the auditory senses. There's a rough > 80% chance that those who once had hearing can hear someone talking over the phone. The chance to use the phone for those who get the implant very early in life is even higher.

We then continue, testing to determine a comfortable volume for each electrode. When complete, all electrodes are activated.

At this point, the patient can hear complete sounds. The wonder, the surprise, and the utter shock of discerning this new sense shows throughout their entire face. It's a difficult moment to articulate. I struggle to explain what it's like to watch a child see their parents say, "I love you" for the first time and hear those tender words rather than simply watching their parent's mouth move. I'm unceasingly mesmerized simply by how visible the impact such a moment is.

After this initial hearing comes an education period, one in which patients must adjust to living with this new sense. They start experiencing with their newfound ability to sense the world and their speech begins to develop. From there, they can begin forming words and piecing them together into coherent sentences. It normally takes a patient about a year to build up a useable understanding of language, an empowering experience, as some of them have not had that ability in their life—unable to convey thoughts, feelings, and emotions through speech.

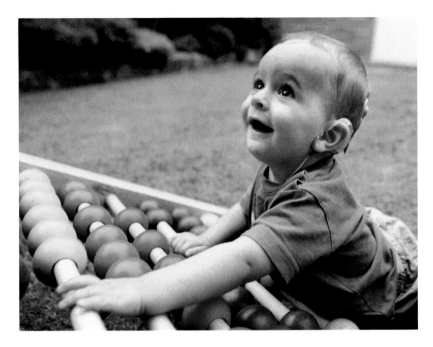

*When a cochlear implant is activated,
deaf children's hearing is born.*

This entire process—of going from deafness to hearing—is incredibly emotional. I try to imagine the feelings parents grapple with. Their child, in some cases their only child, has a disability they do not and because they cannot fully relate, they cannot fully empathize with them. Others struggle with denial: "What do you mean my child is deaf?" and "Surely, not my child" are common sentiments. They eventually accept their inability to fully empathize, and that, perhaps, pains them the greatest. The realization that they're powerless to alleviate this for the beloved child they brought into the world is a heaviness even I, and I'm sure many others, haven't experienced.

Try to imagine going your whole life, or at least a large part of it, without one of your five senses. Imagine you did not know you were missing anything that entire time, that you never knew what it was like be void of the sense of hearing, seeing, touching, tasting, or smelling.

When I do implants, I sometimes wonder what my patients are undergoing. I try to grasp what life without a sense would be like, to, at least in part, empathize with my patients—unaware or unable to change the fact that their experience of the world around them is dampened, muted. But then they are suddenly struck with the great beauty a new sense allows them to perceive. It's a blessing I have never experienced in the way they will.

For most parents, the joy of this moment is a powerful counterweight to any grief they may have previously experienced, for they can now watch their child, the one they birthed and love more than life itself, walk into a new light, into an exciting, fresh breath of life.

In the same way, as a follower of Jesus, I was given a newness of life when I received God himself to live in my heart, and my name was etched into the Lamb's Book of Life. Just as these children hear a sound and engage in a new way to communicate, so we who receive salvation in Christ are led by the Holy Spirit—a new counselor, interpreter, and voice. Through him, God speaks in and through us. It's a completely new experience, a new sense, a new way of living that not only changes our lives but the lives of those around us.

Hard stats dictate that, aside from some irregular exceptions, a single deaf person costs American taxpayers approximately one million dollars. I don't say this to devalue deaf people—assigning a monetary amount to humans definitely does—but to paint an accurate picture not only of the social services required to support a deaf person but how difficult it is for them to live a regular life. In short, helping someone hear benefits society as a whole.

I believe my work has more than just social implications but spiritual ones as well. In many ways, I see the restoration of hearing as a fulfillment of prophecy. Isaiah 35:5 reads, "Then the eyes of the blind will be opened and the ears of the deaf unstopped." As a physician, I feel blessed to be caught in this beautifully miraculous collision of science and technology.

Aside from enhancing the quality of life for an individual, restoration of hearing fulfills another need I believe our Maker instilled in us humans—community. Hearing doesn't just benefit someone as an individual, but it's a gift meant to be shared and one that blesses not just one, but many. Few things connect and bind people together like being able to communicate, and the greater their communication, the tighter the bond. Those who can hear develop language, and the reach of that power is immense.

Before I finish turning an implant on, I ask the patient's parents what is the first thing they want to tell their child. Nearly every time, their message of choice is, "I love you." Yes, sign language can serve as a substitute for speech, but what better conveys the father's love than hearing those three words?

2

A Father's Look

2004

I SAT, IN A SMALL, OLD PERUVIAN HOSPITAL ROOM across the table from a family of three. Father and mother sat abreast their son, flanking the deaf and bewildered, barely three-year-old boy. My purpose was to explain the impending surgery clearly. Through a translator, it was obvious how badly they wanted their son to have this life-changing technology and opportunity. The scene touched me as I saw parents who were considering putting their trust and precious child in my care. It made me want to be worthy of their trust.

This boy was close to his parents, and they with him. They showed it clearly, nonverbally; the concerned glances they aimed toward him when he wasn't looking back at them, their hands clenched around his own, their smiles of gratitude juxtaposed with furrowed brows of concern. They clearly loved their son dearly, and he them. He looked at them (particularly his father) constantly, with trusting glances in place of words, which was his way of asking them to interpret the world around him. They were, to him, his lifeline to the confusing environment around him. Despite his age and disability, he was remarkably adept at understanding their limited communication, void of any words or sign language.

We'd discussed the surgery, how long it would take the boy to hear after it was complete, and how much pain he would endure (fortunately a minimal amount, controllable with medication for a day or two). He was one of 10 patients from just over 200 candidates ranging from age two to four. Five percent. Doesn't sound like much ... does it?

It is, however, quite a load when their surgeries take around two and a half hours each. And we only had two days. They weren't financially positioned to afford a cochlear implant, which is normally an expensive medical device and surgery. For them, this was a narrow window of opportunity. But their gratefulness, like that any other parent, myself included, was mixed with a sense of caution.

I would be drilling into their son's head to make both incisions and insertions in areas of the body where irreparable membranes and other tissues lay. I was confident and skilled in my work, but I can't blame them for being nervous. I would be if it were my own child—even as comfortable as I am with this procedure.

I had experience in hundreds of these surgeries. My goal was to teach local surgeons to perform this delicate micro-surgical procedure so they could serve their patients as the first Cochlear Implant Center in Peru. These would be the first cochlear implants placed in this part of South America. And although I was armed with years of experience, performing surgeries in Peru contrasted mightily with my experience in the United States, the greatest difference being the watertight process that helps us ensure sterilization.

In my usual practice in the United States at a world-renowned medical center, before stepping into the operating room, patients stop by a desk or administration area where they sign a consent form and all the myriad pieces of paperwork required by our system. This process is designed to ensure each patient understands the risks, benefits, alternatives, and complications of their course of action, and to ensure they are acting of their own free will and are of sound mind.

Surgeons usually spend a short time here with their patients in the United States and then leave for the operating room (OR) as others complete the process. Their 'John Hancock' in ink, nurses lead them to a pre-op area (doctor talk for pre-operation). Here, the patients don the oft-dreaded open-backed gown and receive the less dreaded IV and sedation. This is also where the patients' family and friends have a final opportunity to say goodbye and wish their loved one well. From there, anesthesia takes the patient to the OR where the Surgical Team awaits. In the US, this is where surgeons see their patients enter the room on a rolling bed called a gurney.

I know it seems rather cruel to separate family and friends like that, but it's not. It's not our intent to appear cold or distant with the family of patients, particularly parents. We just don't want a space that must stay clean to become contaminated. Clothing can contain germs foreign to our sterile environment, which, in turn, could expose our patients to infection. We take no chances, often bathing the OR, its occupants, as well as the hallway leading to it, in disinfectant.

The protocol in Peru was different. Although the sanitary standards weren't entirely abhorrent, this precaution—of barring parents from taking their child directly into the operation room—contrasted directly with the standards of the US, where parents could be seen in the OR about as often as an extinct animal in the wilderness. Here in Peru, parents carried their children to the door of the OR and literally handed them over to the surgical team. But I didn't know that yet.

On this day, I was preparing early in the morning for the first surgical list with five children waiting their turn in pre-op. I milled about in the OR, prepping my equipment, double checking and, like a pilot, triple checking a checklist—only mine was mental, as is the case for most surgeons. Mission critical equipment—did it make the trip? Is it working? Will it perform when I need it? The fact there is no second chance for these children seemed to add weight to the process. Scalpels, implant kits, all the tools I used for my work, lay awaiting use in neat rank and file.

To understand my heart and the reasons for my actions in ORs like this, I should tell you I have always had a dream—and it goes like this: An old man is sitting at home mulling over his life (that would be me) with his physical prime long past and memories remaining. A knock at the door stirs him to answer it. A smiling young adult greets him and asks, "Do you know who I am?" "No," he says.

The stranger says "I am ___, and you put a cochlear implant in me many years ago when I was young in a far-away country. Because of your willingness, I have learned that my Maker gave me this gift so I could learn to talk and live a normal life. I learned that I am made to serve others and the gift of my hearing is a critical part of my life. I have worked hard, and now I am a teacher, executive, therapist, etc." The old man smiles, and his heart is satisfied.

As the chief physician in Peru, I also played the role of team captain—Captain of the Ship, some call it. I ran through plans with my team, pouring over charts and files, discussing the process by which we'd execute the staircase of procedures that lay between us and an ascension toward a successful implant. Everything was expressed out loud and translated for the benefit of our multiple surgeon trainees.

For some of them, this was their first example of ear surgery. Others had completed similar procedures and had skills that could be built upon to learn this new procedure in only ten cases. I would be taking them through a learning process so they could perform the surgery after I had departed while carrying the teaching to their successors.

In addition, we checked our contingency plans—measures we'd implement if something unexpected reared up during our work. It rarely happens during a cochlear implant, but we planned for the rare. With my dream levitating somewhere in my unconscious I did not want to go home with anything less than a complete success for each of these children.

The discussions continued, the staff shooting questions as I shot back answers. My nurse, who'd worked with me before, helped with the teachings too. I trusted her, and we had a critical working relationship. My trust had been solidified from numerous successful surgeries she'd assisted me in. I needed her as a pilot needs a reliable mechanic who understands his or her preferences, techniques, and methods. She added smoothness and success and reduced my stress and let me focus on the important things—things that bleed.

After our OR pre-surgery prep session was complete, I gave the staff the go-ahead to bring our patient in. But instead of bringing them into the room, they motioned for me to come look down the hall. Still unaccustomed to Peruvian hospital protocol, I obeyed. And there, in that white hallway illuminated by the harsh white light cast by fluorescents, was the father I had met with the night before walking toward me. His arms cradled his treasure, the young boy who looked to him as the interpreter of the world, of his world. Their eyes, both deep and brown, were locked. He clung to his father, who was trying to comfort him, to tell him he'd be ok.

For parents from across the world, children are an equalizer. They render financial and social status irrelevant. I have met rich and poor parents, and the former possess no more ability to heal their child on their own than do the latter. And when a child's health is staked at a crossroads at which danger looms, or where there's even a remote possibility it may, both rich and poor wholly center their concern on their little one. We are all alike in this, in my experience.

People die in surgery, and it happens more often—far more often—in places where physicians use obsolete medical technology. Operating rooms are almost always frightening places, but especially in developing nations. The hallway outside that room could be the last place some families and friends see the ones they love alive. The man had tension holding his son seemingly watching the powerful waves and potentially devastating risk pounding the shoreline of tremendous relief and blessing.

Comforting a child who can hear you can be more than a challenge; this is even more true with deaf children. You can't explain to them what's happening, you can't sing them back to sleep, and you can't assure them they're going to be all right with words. If their parents are present, the children typically look to them, the only thing of familiarity in a room filled with what must, to them, appear unfamiliar and terrifying—people in white coats, carrying around metal instruments, computers blinking, strange sounds, strange smells. I can only imagine how bewildering this scene was to that young boy.

As the father reached the threshold of the OR, the gravity in the sequence of what happened next struck me like a Mac truck:

- Son looks into the room and then at father with a look of uncertainty and fear searching for reassurance.
- Father musters the courage I am sure was not his most pressing feeling and calmly and

gently reassures his deaf son with smiling eyes.
- Father moves his eyes as he nods toward me and son's eyes follow and find mine
- Son looks back at his father and father nods to his son and places his boy in my arms, all the while gazing into my eyes, conveying the trust he was placing, literally, into my hands. Here, he was giving a stranger, one he'd only met once, from a foreign land his most beloved treasure, his flesh and blood and centerpiece of adoration.
- Surgeon looks at father who returns a priceless expression of trust.
- Son puts his arms around my shoulders and goes with me into the OR without so much as a whimper.

Words weren't uttered (we didn't speak the same languages) nor were they needed.

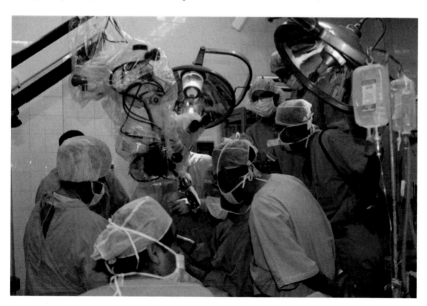

It went perfectly.

There are a few, fleeting moments some of us experience—short, glancing blows of time in which, despite their suddenness and shortness, we see people and undergo a change or shift. These moments touch us in deep, intricate places, places beyond the reach of medicine—the soul—our thoughts, our will, and our emotions. We are as incapable of stopping their reverberations inside us as we are unable to outrun a hungry lion or dam the Mississippi with nothing more than a bucket. They make our lives and become part of us, never to be lost.

I have had a few of these moments, only a handful. They have moved me, sometimes gently, and other times, violently. And they have made me see life and people around me differently. I had one of those moments when that father entrusted his boy to my care.

Following surgery, we placed the boy on the gurney, ready to roll to the recovery room. He breathed heavily, sedated and resting. I felt immense satisfaction, knowing I had done my utmost to give this child a better life. Per protocol, we bandaged him in an inner layer of white gauze, completing the dressing by applying a specially made purple adhesive tape to the outside.

It's a special measure our organization takes for our patients after surgery. For us it's a symbolic gesture—the deep purple reminds us of the color given to royalty as described by God in the Old Testament. Purple is strangely the hardest color to find this material in, but I consider it a necessary symbol of why we do what we do— to remind ourselves and our patients that, to us, they are royalty; they are creatures who, like us, are made in the image of God and are of incalculable value. This father's love is forever seared into my heart as a tangible example of the love from a Father to a child.

A short gurney ride later, he was in the children's recovery room. We stood by him for a few minutes while the anesthesia wore off. I went off in search of his parents and found them in a waiting room. There they waited anxiously to hear of the results and to see their son again. I caught the father's eyes as I walked in. I only had to relay "all is well" with a gentle smile and with my eyes. No words were exchanged. He rose like a shot, as did his wife, without a word, and followed me to the recovery room where their son was waking.

When we arrived after silently walking 100 feet or so, the boy began stirring out of his rest. I could only speculate about the questions running through these parent's heads. Is it him? Is he alive? Is he awake? Does he recognize me? Is he acting normally? Is he actually healed? His parents were glued to his side, embracing him.

The father stayed close, intently watching his beloved while the mom let off steam with rapid words and elation. Shortly, the boy's glances brought the assurance his dad needed. Unable to pick him up off the gurney (we require the patients to stay lying down for a while, even after they have woken) the man bent over, held the child's head, and kissed him repeatedly. He looked at me, a mighty "thank you," rode his gaze, and tears simultaneously welled in both our eyes. That sort of connection comes with working in medicine.

Years passed. I performed hundreds, if not thousands, of implants in other hospitals in other countries around the world and at home. One day, I received a video. "Hello," said a figure on my computer screen. "My name is Jose." I looked closer and recognized him as the Peruvian child whose father had shown me so much trust and gratitude.

The boy, now a few years older, had worked hard to speak both English and Spanish—it's a tough learning process for children born deaf—and proudly showed this newfound form of communication, speaking in both languages with short, simple sentences, sharing his story and how he'd learned to speak. His verbiage was plain and crystal clear, proof positive the implant had been successful. For me and for those who funded his implant, the video is a special treasure.

As a physician, I have found myself shouldering the privilege of providing services for people in desperate need. Every vocation, from gutter cleaning to financial advising, has this same privilege. Those who work in medicine have the privilege of standing in the gap and performing services that not only change lives but sometimes save them. It's given me the chance to see fathers and mothers holding the thing they love most—frequently in tender gratitude—as I did in that Peruvian hospital.

Watching a father embrace his child while letting his emotions pour forth freely and unhindered strikes me with a sort of beauty I haven't witnessed elsewhere on this planet. I think it's the most precious image in the world because—to me—it reflects God's love for humans; it's an image of our heavenly father's relationship with those who call him Abba.

3

Would You Just Die?

1988

IN MEDICAL SCHOOL, we'd worked hard. It felt as though our studies consumed us—consumed our lives, our time, our priorities. Our subjects had a constant hold on the forefront of our thoughts. You're fighting weariness, anxiety, and trying to reach graduation with high marks so you have a good shot at getting a good Residency afterward. And that still isn't enough for some people; not all students end up with the Residency program they hoped for, much fewer good jobs.

Fortunately, I made it to graduation with good marks.

My first year out of medical school, I worked as an intern. As for my fellow graduates, I had enlisted myself in the program to secure a good job. For those of us who thought med school was hard but that we'd passed the worst of it, we were wrong.

It was a trying time, not just for myself, but for other graduates. The load was heavy, even crushing; we worked 100, sometimes 120 hours a week. We could handle it, for the most part, but our main battle became one with sleeplessness.

Mustering amounts of strength that, at times, felt inhuman, we pushed through, taking on responsibilities which the 24 hours in a day didn't provide us enough time to complete (so it seemed).

We worked in a hospital. At night, we were assigned to on-call standby for certain areas. My area was a service surgical center and an intensive care unit. It took up an entire floor. Although the ICU contained only 5 to 10 patients, the rest of the floor held anywhere from 30 to 40.

If a need arose, I would get a call. It could be anything from clarification about a medication or someone having a cardiac arrest. Regardless, I had to stay alert enough to respond with speed and professionalism, neither of which pair well with sleeplessness.

Other interns were assigned to other areas, each with roughly the same amount of work.

And to compound our already crushing load, we worked on teams with people in anywhere from their first to seventh year of training and veteran attendants in their 30s, 40s, 50s, and even 60s. In short, we were grunts at the bottom of a tall ladder.

During this grinding chunk of my life, one of long, sleepless nights, I recall one evening in particular.

The day had been a busy one. So was the evening that followed. I had barely caught a chance to use the restroom and eat. Some days, I didn't; that wasn't abnormal, proof of the busyness of the position.

Four or five months before, I had started the program bright-eyed and bushy-tailed. Now I was hungry and tired and weary. Like marathon runners who break down at the 18-mile mark, I had hit a wall, as do many other interns four or five months in.

I sat there in my on-call room as the clock ticked on somewhere past 2 or 3 a.m. I couldn't sleep. There was one patient on the floor in an unstable condition and another in the ICU faring worse who—suffering from a life-threatening condition—required constant care I had to attentively direct.

In those days we carried a pager that made a swishing beeping sound when patients needed our attention. We'd respond to the call, and they would use it to speak to us. It was basically a one-way radio. The patient in the ICU had called me about six times already that night.

Sometime in the early morning blackness, I had stumbled—still carrying my beeper—out to my car, attempting to snatch a few moments of sleep. I wasn't neglecting my post; things had just gotten quiet. I had gone down hard and quick, as you'd expect for someone running on too little sleep. In about three minutes, I was sleeping deeply.

What I recall being the ICU patient's seventh call that night shattered my rest. Utter misery, it seemed, was my portion that night. My eyes were burning, pulling in and out of focus constantly, and it was hard to keep them open. The building containing the ICU unit was probably 300 yards away from my car. Slowly, I got up, opened the door, and stepped into the night air. My joints, stiff with weariness, tightened, resisting. I hated being awake. I hated being that tired.

"Would you just die?" I sullenly muttered.

My words shocked me, so subtle, yet so foreign to my vocabulary, to my usual thoughts. It was as though someone else had said them. I was taken aback by the utter lack of empathy, the utter ruthlessness of them.

I just told a patient to die. That's cold, so opposite of why I signed on the dotted line to become a doctor.

That moment rooted me down in my thoughts, forcing me to reflect on my own heart. In that moment, I had crossed the threshold of my stamina—some people refer to it as "reaching the end of yourself"—my breaking point. I got a raw, unfiltered glimpse of the lack of empathy, sacrificial love, and ability to handle a difficult situation with grace. It was overwhelming and quite sad—an epiphany many in the medical experience have experienced.

For about 30 seconds, I stood by my car, facing off with my own heart. Then I trudged forth to do what I had been trained to and assisted the ailing man.

At first, the situation didn't change. For the three or four days following that night, his continual calls for assistance persisted—the swooshing beep became a steady constant. But despite the ongoing circumstances, something in me had begun to change. I could feel it.

Looking back, I realize that my revelation in the parking lot that night during my internship was, in fact, a gift in disguise. It provided me a chance to reflect and take in a humbling, painful dose of conviction. And I'm glad it hurt; better to feel pain—even if it's birthed from regret or guilt—than remain callous to conscious and truth.

After the harsh realization I had that late night, I adjusted my attitude. Yes, I still had a lot of growing to do, and I knew that, but my disposition had shifted. I was determined to keep him going and attended to him constantly. I pushed through the fatigue, placing his need over my own. It was hard, but I knew it was right and that I couldn't face my heart like I had in that parking lot if I didn't do what was right. It was hard work, but I was held by a convicting determination to keep him alive.

In the end, the patient survived and, after a few more days of care, was released from the hospital.

"You're not going to die," I had told him before he turned for the better; sure enough, he didn't.

Meanwhile, I had learned to live more humbly and effectively as a physician.

4

Caitlin's Fall

1989

PARENTS OF DEAF CHILDREN express a wide range of emotions: fear, anger, helplessness, and others. Really, every parent to a child with critical needs probably feels them. I have seen them expressed in waiting rooms, preoperating rooms, in American hospitals with the first world's best technology, and in dirt-floored clinics of small, jungle nations. I can recognize them, sniff them out. And not just because I have worked with parents, but because I am one.

I fell in love with Julia, the woman I married, when I was a junior in college. We dated for a just over a year and, a week after we completed undergraduate school, gave our vows. A few weeks more and I began the all-encompassing task of medical school. My preverbal plate, I thought, couldn't get fuller. I was wrong; Julia and I were blessed with a pregnancy. On June 7, 1985, I held our newly birthed daughter Caitlin Crist Roberson. She was born on the first day of my pediatrics rotation—the first time I had been in the clinic after two grueling years of textbook-based learning and memorization. Time flew during that wonderful time.

A couple of years drifted by, which felt like months. By then, I had become a budding surgeon after graduating from medical school and entering residency training. Finally, I was able to get beyond the general and broad education of medical school to experience the many different subspecialties of surgery. I loved my work and interacting with patients.

Each rotation took me to a new service: thoracic surgery, vascular surgery, trauma surgery, etc. At the time of this story, I was a Resident in the hospital Emergency Room. In our grueling 24-hour shifts, we treated an array of patients—hard work, but good work. Despite the demanding schedule, I had more time to spend with Julia and Caitlin than usual since other rotations were more of a "40 hours on / 8 hours off" arrangement.

I loved those days. Some were spent with hikes and stroller walks, others, in our apartment on the third floor of a housing unit for medical students, marked with an occasional ride on our motorcycle to the local ice cream parlor. Julia got pregnant again, and a second baby was on its way. Life was demanding, exciting, and just plain good.

One weekend during this blissful season, I fell sick—like I had caught something from the emergency room or hospital. The vomit didn't wait long to make an entrance. Not wanting Julia, who suffered from pregnancy sickness, to encounter the rank odor now lingering in our bathroom, I opened a floor-to-ceiling window.

The day, until then, had been a happy one of easy resting. I had read a devotional book to Caitlin and taught her John 16:33. Then Caitlin, Julia, and I went hiking in a local garden. It was a new world for our little girl, filled with new sights, sounds, a world of trees and leaves and creatures—squirrels and frogs specifically.

A river ran alongside us for some time. Dogs, sometimes horses and their riders, came by. Caitlin adored the horses, squealing with excitement and pointing at them upon approach. We sat in the grass by the river for some time, munching on the picnic of ham and cheese sandwiches and oranges. Caitlin had apple juice and two of the cookies she'd helped Julia bake.

We tossed some rocks into the river before hiking back up to the main trail. Passing horseback riders halted and let Caitlin pet their mounts, Strawberry and Travis. Caitlin thought it was funny a creature that so dwarfed her was named Strawberry. When she petted them, their manes tickled her, and she laughed, smiling—as she had the entire adventure—reveling in a pure, childlike joy, at life and its goodness.

I knew leaving the window open was dangerous. A friend of ours lost their child, Kelly, to complications resulting from a fall out of a first-floor window. Julia and I had agreed to take precautions against a similar incident.

I'll let Julia know, I told myself. After all, she was sick, and that smell was, well, I'll let your imagination figure that out. In short, I didn't want her to get sicker. She was napping and yielding to the weakness the sickness caused, and I soon was as well, with Caitlin following suit, lying on my chest. I was too tired and too sick to worry.

"She's fallen! She's fallen out the window!"

I could hear Julia yelling, her words jolting me out of the blackness of sleep. I checked my watch; less than an hour had ticked by.

"Caitlin! Caitlin!" Julia screamed from the bathroom. I ran to the window, afraid of what I would see. The screen was torn, the underwear from Caitlin's dolly on the floor, and Julia was screaming. I felt sick, not with the nausea of a stomach bug or the flu, but a heavy, clogged feeling down deep in my gut. It was hard to breathe. "She's fallen out the window! Out the window!" my wife shouted.

I looked out the opening and down, and there she was on the hard, burnt orange clay, lying unconscious and still, just as she'd been on my chest a few hours before.

I was helpless—at least I felt so. The anguish is almost indescribable. I couldn't think, I couldn't rationalize or process what'd happened. The moments afterward were a blur. I found myself flying down the staircase, sprinting around the building. Falling to my knees, I swept my daughter up in my arms, holding her.

"What are you doing?" screamed Julia, rounding the building in succession. "Why did you pick her up?"'

I was frozen. That she had just fallen—instead of falling a long time ago as I assumed—fallen at least 30 feet, struck me hard when my wife posed the question.

Is she alive? I asked myself. *Did I cause further damage, maybe even paralyze her when I picked her up?*

Later, I remembered the piece of clothing from Caitlin's dolly, and the whole thing made sense. Recently, she'd made it a point to try to put her doll's clothes on herself. Big enough to slip over her foot, but too small to go up her leg, it must have entangled her. Hearing her mother in the bathroom, she probably wandered in to find her, only to find the window open, a new sight to her that would snag the curiosity of any two-year-old. The underwear tripped her as she trod across the slippery linoleum bathroom floors. The vinyl screen—the only thing separating her from the outside—couldn't halt her and tore when she fell into it.

Julia confirmed it all. She'd seen it happen, watched from too far away to intervene.

In the momentary haste to reach her, the obvious had eluded me, and now the reality fell hard. Caitlin could be dead.

Julia, armed with sharp, motherly wisdom, swooped in, her calm intuition blocking the crippling despair that could have otherwise rendered us insensible and incapacitated.

"You have been trained. You know what to do," she said. "Just do it."

The doctor in me—the quick-thinking, confident physician who'd been sharpened by years of work in an emergency room—took control. I was in automatic mode now. No time to worry; no time to reflect; no time to regret, or cry or fear—just procedures, a plain, straightforward set of steps. I knew them intuitively; they were second nature, branded in me by years of schooling. They were muscle memory. All I had to do was keep moving, which now mattered more than any moment in my career. Maybe the hours I had spent away from my daughter in a hospital would save her.

"Call an ambulance," I coolly ordered Julia while checking Caitlin's pulse. A pulse emanated from tiny arteries in her tiny wrists, though feeble. She wasn't breathing for herself.

Mouth to mouth brought no response.

Please God, please give my daughter life.

I try again, nothing.

Again, nothing.

And again, nothing.

Again, nothing, heart sinking.

A minute ticks off, then another as I breathe for her. And then, a breath—a single shallow breath—not enough to sustain her but at least an effort. Still no consciousness, but at least a ray of hope—no, a breath of hope. Back to mouth to mouth. A few tries, and then she's breathing more deeply. We cry to her, "breath! Breathe!" but she can't. I have to keep giving her mouth-to-mouth though. If I don't, she can't.

A small crowd had formed, mostly neighbors. They watched, nervously and concerned. Police had arrived to, the lights from their cars casting a red and blue and purple show of lights about. A few minutes later, an ambulance arrived, whisking Caitlin and me away to the hospital. Julia followed in a police car. During the ride, I alternated with an EMT to keep Caitlin breathing.

I was the first one out of the vehicle when we reached the emergency room. Everything, the beds, equipment, machinery, instrumentation, even the staff, was in the proper order, rank, and file I had grown accustomed to. It brought somewhat of a calmness. I called my fellow residents forth and informed them of the situation. I was flipping between a trained professional and a father with a more than a broken heart.

A part of me felt in control, only now the patient was my daughter, not a stranger—I had seen plenty of them, dozens some nights. So even though everything looked the same, sounded the same, smelled the same, remained at its usual post, this was entirely different. Even the colleagues who I had relied on for their professional medical work, I, along with my wife and Caitlin, now depended on in an intimate, personal way.

Our daughter woke slightly while in the ER but then lost consciousness again.

The residents and other hospital staff stuck a breathing tube down Caitlin's throat and x-rayed her chest and spine from the front and side and put a C-collar around her neck. They started IVs and turned oxygen on too and began blood tests and further examinations.

Julia and I waited in the family holding area in the ER while the controlled chaos of the trauma room went on with my firstborn as the focus. The story of Kelly loomed in our minds. One fourth, her fall was one fourth the distance of Caitlin's fall. I know the knowledge I had of medicine saved Caitlin's life, but at this point, the knowledge of what could have happened and what could be happening to end her life or maim her beautiful little body seemed almost like a curse.

The pain of losing Caitlin seemed too heavy, yet possibly a likely outcome. I know the statistics of death and permanent disability from falls in children. Agony, that's what it was, but on a level I had never felt before—never in an OR, or an ER, or in any other situation, medical or non-medical. We prayed for God to heal her, or if she wasn't to be healed, that He'd take her home to heaven. The gravity of a permanently disabled family member and its effect on our marriage and our lives was too much to even think about.

Amid our waiting and praying, there had been one glimmer of comfort. Caitlin had woken for a moment and seemed to recognize her surroundings. It indicated the possibility that her brain had not been so injured in the fall that she would never regain consciousness. Our friends had trickled in soon after our arrival at the hospital, praying with and for us. Even hospital staff we knew—Bret, Marlene, and Doug and Barbie—offered comfort through both words and their presence.

Julia and I kept waiting. My status as father and husband kept me out of the world, out of the perspective of a medical practitioner working with fully objective judgment. My experience as a surgeon tore away the comforting veil of ignorance to hospital practices so many parents enjoy. The somber faces of my peers who cared for her and who came by to offer comfort were perhaps the scariest reality to face, as they all knew, as I did, how serious this was.

I was like a ghost, trapped between two worlds, anxiously moving between the second floor (where Caitlin was admitted in ICU) and fifth floor (where Julia was admitted to get IV fluids to protect the child she was carrying) for seventy-two hours; it was excruciating. I would have walked through fire—literally—to help both of them, to alleviate their pain, to bring them comfort or hope or joy, and here I was confined to the sidelines, to watch and not play. I am not a good "watch and wait" type of guy.

Caitlin had suffered a severe concussion, which warranted CT scans. Her spleen was ruptured. Her skull was fractured. The left lung had a large bruise within it, indicating the force of her fall. Her ribs were broken, as was her left wrist. Fortunately, her spine and abdominal area seemed ok, which isn't usually the case for patients who experience forceful impacts like hers.

And although some of the staff thought the scans indicated she'd fractured her femur, an orthopedic surgeon, upon examining the slide, ensured us her femur was all right. A large blood clot was present in her left thigh. There was also what appeared to be blood between the brain and the inner portion of the skull. That is usually bad news, as permanent brain damage is associated with the finding. I was in the anteroom of the scanner when the images appeared on the screen, and I knew exactly what they showed. It was a punch in the gut and the most disastrous finding, as I knew all the other injuries would heal.

As the splenic tear was small, at least at this time no trip to the OR would be necessary.

Hours later, I was wearing a rut in the floor down the floor of the hospital's ICU. Caitlin was here, recovering, attended to by people I considered co-workers. One of them was Sonya, the wife Gary, a fellow resident who was a neurosurgeon. I was thankful Sonya was there. An experienced neurosurgery nurse—particularly pediatric neurosurgery—Sonya watched and monitored Caitlin throughout her first night there as I continued to come in and out of the room.

Three floors above me, Julia rested as well. Although we'd checked on Julia regularly through the night, she was dehydrated and sick from her pregnancy and going on little to no sleep. She'd been overcome by exhaustion and admitted by the hospital. I didn't leave her side without promising I would do everything in my human power to make sure Caitlin got the best care.

Caitlin didn't respond to stimulation the first night. The next morning, Julia and I scrambled down to see her. She was still unresponsive due to the necessary sedation given to allow the brain swelling to be treated. It was disappointing but understandable. We returned to our rooms, holding to hope but feeling grim.

After waiting many more hours and haunting the halls of the hospital, I took another of my innumerable trips downstairs. Since Julia had to rest, I went alone. I have no memory of what time of the day or night it was, as that had no meaning to me. Her sedation had been eased, and the following days would allow us to tell how much damage had been done. The ventilator was still breathing for her through the tube inserted into her breathing passage.

As before, I started speaking to Caitlin, only this time, those sweet little eyes opened as I talked. My heart was filled with encouragement. I knew she not only had a better chance of survival but of retaining her mental health and strength. I rushed upstairs to Julia with the welcomed news, kissing and caressing her. However, by the time we got downstairs, Caitlin had fallen into unresponsiveness. Again, we returned upstairs.

About forty-five minutes after her first response, I checked on her, and she responded again, holding and even squeezing my hand. Again, I brought Julia down to an unresponsive Caitlin. It was hard for her to hear about her daughter's recovery but be unable to witness it. But later that morning while Julia was present, Caitlin responded a third time, glancing about the room, still dazed as though she were looking past us. As the day progressed, she continued responding, and though she couldn't talk because of the endotracheal and nasogastric tube, she improved with each passing hour. The third time she looked at me and mouthed the word, "Papa." I think I took the first deep breath of the past three days or more.

On Monday, her second night in the hospital, Caitlin was able to nod. I had asked her if she wanted to see her mommy, and she indicated yes by nodding. I was still anxious though. If an edema—an uncontrollable injury that takes down the parts of the brain controlling vital functions—developed, it could kill her in a matter of hours. I kept close tabs, as did a host of other residents, doctors, and medical students—John Gartman, Gary Powell, Dr. Powers, and interns Doug Wilson and Jeff Tomkins. There was also the pediatric surgery service, Charles Miller, and Dr. Lacey. And those were just a few. Many of my personal friends made sure to look out for us, specifically Julia and Caitlin. My colleagues even took on-call responsibilities so I could be with my wife and child, and the surgery department told me to take as much time off as I needed.

The window for the edema to manifest came and went, and I breathed yet another heavy sigh of relief. And then, more good news—the CT scan that had originally seemed to show a subarachnoid hemorrhage was nothing more than glitchy software, the Radiologist explained. There was no subarachnoid hemorrhage. However, radiologists were concerned over what they thought could be a fracture at the apex of the cervical spine, a fracture that could cause so much instability in Caitlin's neck that it could dislocate instantly; that would, in turn, cause paralysis and death. But further analysis on a hospital computer showed that, as before, it was the CT scan, not Caitlin, that had the problem; there was no fracture.

The only problem that really turned out to be a problem was Caitlin's arm. After some swelling, staff x-rayed it and found a slight fracture. Requiring a cast instead of requiring only a splint, the injury revealed that she'd extended her arm in front of her to break her fall, a reactionary move that may have saved her life.

That second night, though Caitlin was far from being out of the woods, she'd made some major improvements. Curled up on a reclining chair in Caitlin's room so we could check on her regularly, Julia and I could barely sleep. Julia's IV was a constant reminder of the new life inside her to consider, too. My mind continually turned to the worries and prayers I had felt and uttered during our wait in the emergency room those first few moments after we'd arrived, when everything felt raw. Now I felt that perhaps Caitlin would be ok. As a physician, I had seen plenty of patients take a turn for the worse. That made me keep my hopes down. But now it seemed Caitlin would be ok.

My family was in rough shape—Caitlin, a two-year-old in a C-Collar, and Julia, pregnant, sick, and dehydrated. But things were looking hopeful. God, in His loving mercy, had kept our girl alive and given her the prospect of recovering to live a happy, healthy life. I'm happy to say she's had just that. Although her injuries could have caused anything from something as minor as a concussion to permanent disabling traumatic brain injury, Caitlin survived with no lasting damage. And because of that, I'm so thankful for those who came together in prayer.

I was told that our friends and we weren't the only ones praying for Caitlin. A family friend called some friends and loved ones, who in turn reached out to believers they knew. It was a wildfire that spread so that in a matter of hours, two churches and their congregations, as well as somewhere between 300 and 350 workers at a Billy Graham convention, took to their knees in prayer for Caitlin. I valued prayer like never before after that.

I tell this story to share my experience as not only a doctor or surgeon scientist but as a parent. For years, I had known that parents undergo anxiety when their child is endangered. Living through that—going through a gauntlet of emotions and fears and worries and even joys with Julia—provided me an appreciation for what parents experience that I don't think I would have attained any other way. It's been a story I have told and will always continue to tell—one of the blessings in disguise that strengthened my family, faith in God, and empathy for people. I still don't know what it's like to lose a child, but I hope through that harrowing day years ago, I can better comfort those who have.

Tuesday morning, Caitlin was able to breathe without the help of an endotracheal tube. She was sleepy throughout the rest of the day but grew steadily more alert. In the early afternoon, Julia stepped out of the room. I sat there watching Caitlin, truly hopeful she'd be all right. As I watched, I saw her eyes lock onto something. Turning, I saw Julia re-enter. Caitlin must have recognized her. Caitlin smiled.

Later, she woke from a nap.

"Hi, Papa," she said after she saw me. "I want Mommy."

Her first words to my wife were, "Mommy, I almost fell out a window!"

"Yes, darling girl, you almost did."

By that afternoon, she was out of her bed and in our arms. We bathed her, Julia brushed her teeth, and we showered her with kisses. Later that evening, I stood by her bed as she rested peacefully, hooked into only one machine—an oxygen saturation monitor.

The monitors beeped softly as the machine hummed gently. Caitlin stirred, turned, and fell back into a restful doze, a sight perfect and beautiful to me, a man lucky to be her father.

5

Halt! Who Goes There?

1990

MY WORK, AS YOU HAVE PROBABLY GATHERED, is usually serious, even dangerous. And sometimes that's an understatement. But walking away from some situations, my
greatest concern wasn't for my health or safety, but that I
wouldn't be able to keep a straight face when I thought
about them. This is one of those situations.

As a young surgeon-in-training, I held a position at
the bottom of a totem pole; the newer you are, the more
undesirable your assigned tasks. I had completed four
years of undergraduate schooling, the same of medical
school, but now I had been flung into a bigger pond:
Surgery Residency Training. Although I had completed 8
out of the 15 total years of schooling it would take to become an ear surgeon, here I was so low they simply referred to me as "intern," a title held by all my fellow co-
horts in that bottom tier.

As my position dictated, I had many less-than-
desirable responsibilities—actually, detested might better
describe them. Still, they were necessary—welcome to
one of the early lessons of becoming a surgeon. Most
surgeries on a patient's abdomen, which are performed

by general surgeons, require the patient's bowels to be clear (usually via laxatives, bulk-forming agents like those advertised on television, or enemas) and the inside of the system to be washed with a bacteria-killing solution. Any of this "debris" can cause terrible infections if it contacts an open wound during surgery. Someone must make sure the process is complete and goes well. This was where other interns and I put in some of our most undesirable hours, sometimes late into the night, clearing the decks for tomorrow's surgeries.

One night, I was tending to a tiny little old lady who was due for general surgery the next morning. As part of my job, I was barred from going to bed until I had confirmed all the GI tracts (medical lingo for bowels) of the patients scheduled for surgery the following day had been cleared.

I had gotten through seven or eight patients fairly easily in two or three hours but had reached a roadblock with this frail and regal elderly woman.

Sparing you the details, I'll simply say we'd tried the means provided to clear her GI track, only to no avail. It was about an hour and a half after midnight, and although we were reaching the point of a red-eyed cocktail of despair and misery—including for the patient herself— we couldn't give up.

What she had was life-threatening, and it had to come out. In a few hours, a fresh surgical team would do their best on her behalf. She was tired, I was tired, and so was the staff. If I'm aggravated, I thought, I can't imagine what she's feeling. She'd been through more than a normal person should have to, and at her age, well, I knew I couldn't even begin to relate. Life is tough and at times even cruel, and nowhere can it be more evident than in the wards of a hospital. This example of the human spirit still cheers me to this day.

After leaving her to try to take care of her business for some time in her room, I re-entered a short time later, knocking softly on her door. It was quiet—quiet as only the wee hours of the morning can be. I stepped in, took a step, and then another, listening for any reaction from behind the curtain. I stood for another moment, and then I heard her. In a sweet, frail voice she said, "Halt! Who goes there? Friend or enema?"

6

Rupture

1990

WORKING IN AN EMERGENCY ROOM can be an exercise in extremes. Emergency rooms and their staff are frequently the first line of touch for individuals with urgent, time-sensitive medical conditions–it can be an emotionally charged environment. Nonetheless, there are lulls and doldrums–moments of grinding boredom during which it feels like the clock runs off Nyquil instead of batteries–and as any professional with experience in these environments knows well, bursts of wild tempest–action and adrenaline-fueled controlled chaos as patients are brought in at the interface of life and death.

Emergency rooms contain some of the heroes of medicine as staff physicians initiate treatment for potentially lethal conditions, drawing on the entire hospital staff as the needs demand. The injuries and conditions range from minimal to grave–those double sliding doors open and anyone from a lacrosse player with a broken arm, to a police officer whose had rifle rounds punch holes in his chest, may come through; we get the calm, the storm, and everything in between.

Medical training involves undergraduate work for four years (with an emphasis on courses having to do with the human body, such as biology, genetics, physiology, etc.) similar to courses taken by anyone who goes to college. The next four years are medical school. The first two years consist of a demanding classroom schedule featuring in-depth courses on all aspects of human normalcy and pathology. The material is not difficult to understand in concept, but the volume of material is enormous. The next two years of medical school involve rotations in specialties of medicine (such as pediatrics, surgery, psychiatry, and internal medicine) and finally some electives during the fourth year, where candidate MDs can begin to focus their interest.

Next, a residency is selected (this decision is made after the third-year rotations, thereby allowing future physicians to sample areas of medicine and see where they fit), which can last from three to eight years. My training, for example, took 11 years after college. It's a long road but one I would gladly travel again! To put it in focus, when I received my high school diploma, I had more education in front of me than behind me.

As future physicians progress through this schedule, they are granted more responsibility (provided they prove themselves worthy). Most future physicians—and I was no exception—are itching to finally get their experience on an actual patient about six to seven years into their training. After medical school and in residency, residents reach new levels of responsibility. They provide much of the manpower of many teaching hospitals. They are low paid but an important part of health care delivery in the United States.

One story from my residency training left an indelible imprint on me, as it was early in my career. As a senior resident in charge of the emergency room, I crewed this vessel regularly, a responsibility I loved. Being on the front lines made me feel deep inside that I was made for this. I remember the thrill of standing on the landing pad knowing another human was rocketing toward our team after a serious accident, hanging between life and death. It would be up to us to diagnose, stabilize, and restore, backed by the entire hospital of specialists and resources.

I was manning my post late one evening around 11 p.m. with 8 hours of my 24-hour shift to go. Our radio crackled and EMTs (Emergency Medical Technicians who man ambulances) called about an incoming patient. These heads-up calls, typical of EMTs, provide us a few moments to brace for impact and prep for the incoming patient. This particular individual, a college football star and NFL draftee, had been pulled, unconscious, out of what was formerly recognizable as a sports car with less than 500 miles on the odometer; crashing at high speed has that effect on vehicles. It's a common result of the recipe of youth and powerful motors. His vitals (heart rate, blood pressure, etc.) reportedly fluctuated, dipping and rising and then dipping again. He was in serious trouble.

Any lingering calm and quiet shattered as staff rushed to their battle stations, just as we'd rehearsed time and time before with and without patients—just like any special forces group does; nurses running here, doctors there, a perfectly organized frenzy of white coat and scrub-clad professionals dashing about. It would probably severely rattle your nerves., but due to our practice and understanding of everyone's roles, it was poetry in motion to me.

Per the EMT's ETA (estimated time of arrival), the helicopter bearing the patient landed, and the staff, gurney in tow, moved with the seriousness the case mandated. One glance at their body language alone could dismiss even the strongest doubt of their urgency. It is a privilege to experience the feelings you have as a team, where you can trust and depend on others to create an outcome no one could achieve alone!

The landing pad was dark. Our coats flapped about as powerful wind from the mighty mechanical beast descended. It soon touched down (gentler than I expected), and I got my first look at the patient. Despite the lack of lighting, I could see he was indeed in bad shape. He was bloodied all over, and his clothing, rent and torn, a disheartening sight. I think everyone felt something similar in their hearts, and if I had spoken, I think I would have said, "It's up to us people–time to bring everything you have trained for."

With the utmost gentleness, we loaded the young man strapped to a backboard and in a collar around his neck with all the attached monitoring equipment onto the gurney. After a while, you develop a sixth sense when you treat patients, being able to gauge the urgency of the situation. This one was not a drill. We rocketed the gurney inside the hospital and reached the ER trauma room located just off the helipad.

In a trauma room, every conceivable evaluation tool and piece of equipment is organized to allow us to access the things we need within seconds. This kind of logistical preparation can mean the difference between life and death. If a patient needs a tube inserted through the ribs to re-expand their collapsed lung or a transfusion is needed due to severe blood loss, you don't have even a couple of minutes to wait for it to be located and delivered from another room. You need it now.

Our team began the "ABC's," a sort of pre-established survival checklist that urgent care physicians use to prioritize procedures in situations this critical; A means clear airway, B means make sure breathing is ongoing (either by the patient or provided by us), and C means check circulation or blood flow.

We hit our first snag on step A. Although his airway was clear of obstruction, the severity of the impact had rendered his respiratory efforts irregular, so we inserted an endotracheal tube down his throat and into the breathing passage that leads to the lungs. The end outside his body was fixed to a ventilator machine (a sort of artificial lung, pushing and pulling air to and from his lungs) whose low, electric hum may have been oxygen. A and B were instituted. Blood pressure was low but adequate, and a catheter was inserted in an artery to give instantaneous readouts, which we followed continually as a single data point in a sea of changing data.

Though we'd cleared the first steps relatively simply, we were still blind to the extent of his injuries. His chest had taken a heavy blow during the crash, and despite his steady blood pressure, we suspected internal bleeding. To be prepared to respond to a drop in blood pressure, we started an intravenous fluid drip via a catheter inserted in a large vein where the leg meets the torso.

Giving either fluid or blood would serve to refill his tank if the injury caused to leak out so severely that the blood pressure dropped. The staff proceeded to check the patient over, examining joints for further injury, hunting for any lacerations or contusions, and getting x-rays of his cervical and lower spine. A routine sequence was necessary to check everything, as the patient could not respond to us in his unconscious state.

Others, armed with flashlights, examined his eyes and how they reacted to light—a method used for diagnosing concussions. Watching his eyes' reflexes helped them make the call. I'd been hopeful he'd only sustained moderate injuries. He looked pretty roughed up, yes, but I'd seen other patients who looked worse with injuries less severe. He was young, handsome, and had a promising career ahead of him.

The thought of him sidelined before his first NFL season began was sad, but I couldn't allow it to linger; such sentiments can fog the mind of a physician when he needs to think clearly. We try not to get emotionally attached to patients in general, but we're also human. It's a blurry line to walk. In reality, these feelings can only last seconds in the heat of the moment. You move on to answer the pressing question: what is the most immediate threat and what is the total list of injuries we must prioritize?

Meanwhile, an x-ray tech had placed x-ray plates (at this time, they were still the hardcopy, greenish-grey, vinyl screens) in a slot on the gurney underneath the patient—one built specifically for this situation. We snapped images of his head and neck, all the way down his spine, to his pelvis, and simultaneously notified the intensive care unit; regardless of results, we knew he'd probably need more than a few x-rays and bandages. The x-rays had to be processed at that point and developed much like film used to be developed. Now it's instantaneous, as digital images flicker to life on huge monitors in the room.

As a first-line trauma surgeon, it was my responsibility to give the x-rays a first pass and spot anything that appeared abnormal once they returned from processing. A certified radiologist would review them later, but for now, I acted as lookout. At this point, our patient had been in the facility for less than seven minutes.

The first few slides showed nothing of concern, just intact bones, hues, and shades of the murky white marrow—as would be found in a healthy person. I continued sifting through the vinyl, and then I reached the region of the chest. I stopped. Something was off. It was subtle but severe. I double and triple checked in my mind to be completely sure.

Normally, in x-rays of the chest, there's a bulge (shaped like a green onion) created by the aorta—the vessel that carries blood to the body—just above its exit from the heart. If it's functioning properly, delivering the red substance to its proper destination, it'll show up in the image. On this slide, I couldn't spot the bulge—it was a straight tube—a subtle but critical sign. We now had a situation that was about to deteriorate rapidly in the most serious way.

Understand, the upper arch of the aorta is tethered to the chest. It rests in the back of the chest and is secured there by ligaments and connective tissue. It's generally a strong bond. Lower along the curve of the greatest blood vessel in the body where it turns to go to the lower body, this bond is far weaker.

During severe frontal impacts like this young man underwent, it can break loose from these lower bonds while the upper bonds hold. This can create a zone of severe stress where the two segments transition, tearing the artery, unleashing a torrent of blood that floods the chest cavity, leading to instant death. In rare cases, like this one, a partial tear occurs, and blood begins to track its way along the blood vessel back toward the heart, obscuring the bulge I had been looking for on the x-ray. A partial tear can and will turn to a full tear due to the blood pressure behind this "crack in the dam," at any moment killing the patient instantly.

This was a ticking time-bomb of an issue—threat level raised, nurse's and doctor's talking raised to yelling, the former shouting readings on vitals, the latter delivering orders acronymically. In seconds, we grabbed the gurney, now manned by three to four staff on both sides, and whisked it out of the trauma room, thundering down the hallway and into an elevator. The ride was brief but gave me a second to reflect. *Are we going to be fast enough? He could be seconds away from leaving this earth!* The elevator doors opened, we dismounted, and clinging, knuckles white on the metal bars of the cart, sprinted the remaining 800 yards—the distance of eight football fields—to the OR. We burst into the room, heaving for air.

Time was only an enemy at this point; the more spent, the narrower our patient's window of survival grew. Without sterilizing the operative field as we always do in a controlled situation, we lifted the still living, shredded man out of the gurney and onto the OR bed. Unconscious, his breathing tube was connected to the anesthesia machine as medications hastily drawn up into syringes were emptied into his bloodstream to make sure he didn't feel pain or move.

Ignoring formalities to save precious time, a thoracic surgeon (chest surgeon) who was in the hospital met us in the OR. Armed with a large, razor-edged scalpel and a calm, gritty intensity, he opened the patient's chest with an incision starting at the sternum and extending under the arm halfway to the spine, extending between the ribs and into the lung cavity.

As a surgery resident, I served as an assistant working alongside the other team members, clustered around our only focus. After the incision had been made, we widened the incision with a spreader—a type of reverse clamp that forces gaps to stay open. None winced. This is the nature of emergency trauma work. Callous as it may seem, such procedures were usual. Still, there was an added sense of urgency, considering how brutal the injury had been and how it could turn sour so quickly.

The senior thoracic surgeon, having rushed down from his on-call room upstairs to assist us, thrust his arm into the cavity. With swift efficiency, he grabbed the aorta and placed clamps above and below the tear, stemming the blood loss. If he hesitated, we didn't notice.

The first stage had been cleared, but we only let out a half-breath of relief, aware of the body's inability to survive long without blood flow. After the clamp was applied, blood still flowed to the head, arms, and brain, but the major supply to the lower body was now at zero. The crack in the dam had been temporarily patched, but the real problem, the torn aorta, had to be repaired. The clock had started on the time to repair the torn vessel and release the clamps to restore the life-sustaining blood flow from the chest down.

The procedure that followed could be likened to a swift but delicate clock repair (but one that bleeds) deep in a body cavity, with the pressure of time limits to complete your work or a life is lost. I know it sounds a bit weird, but the coordination and intensity of my fellow professionals—individuals whose skill was only rivaled by their own intelligence—was a beautiful thing to watch; only a few are privileged to ever behold it. As they deftly wielded scalpels, needles, scissors, retractors, and other gleaming instruments, you wouldn't notice they battled against time in an orchestra in which no less than 10-15 tasks were performed simultaneously. Above the bed, a clock ominously ticked on, an unceasing reminder of the dreaded window that grew ever narrower; as it did, so increased their earnestness and intensity.

Twenty-four minutes later, it was done; in 24 minutes, the aorta was sewn up and repaired; in 24 minutes, the patient's blood was flowing into his lower body as it should as the clamps were released. The crack in the dam was repaired, and the dam was holding! The surgical team stood, sweating, wet with the perspiration brought about by their immense efforts. They were overwhelmed with the gravity of the situation deep in the morning hours while the town around us slept. It was the first time they'd had a moment to stop since we got that first call from the EMTs.

Amid this hustle, there'd been a constant drone, a ringing of medical terminology. For me, the jargon had become a second language. Now that it had ceased, I noticed not one extraneous word had been spoken that I can recall—only those things which aided the task.

We stood around the patient, who was motionless save for the steady rise and fall of his chest and sound of the breathing machine, and watched, eyeing the monitors. Those dark, glass screens, glowing with red and green pulses on vitals, fed us information on the patient's health, which we subconsciously translated (thanks to our med school education) as we eagerly watched him first settle and then lie stable and resting—blood flow steady, blood pressure holding. The chest remained open, held there by the rib-spreading retractor. Looking inside, you could see places no one was ever meant to see—the pink, glistening, marvelous structures and construction of the human form, now with a neat row of sutures extending completely around the two-inch muscular tube called the aorta as it pulsed with each heartbeat.

I think for the first time in a bit, all our heart rates began to settle toward a normal range. We knew the oncoming train of an aortic rupture had been stopped. The OR, however, was a ridiculously chaotic mess. We lacked the normal-ordered logistics of mono-chromatic drapes walling off the whole of the patient from their wound.

Blood and fluid were all over us, and a massive amount of packaging and supplies and instruments littered the floor and surrounding tables, as we only had time to open and drop the many dozen things we urgently needed. All of us started to restore order by putting things into their normal places, draping the patient and sterilizing parts of the skin around the wound—allowing a few minutes for things to stabilize, including our minds and hearts.

I hope you can get a sense of the teamwork and battle, which goes on silently to the outside world, in some of our nation's ORs. Men and women of incredible courage, fortitude, and action inhabit them. One analogy is that of a sports team (in this case, we were definitely the underdog!) lining up against an adversary. After the game is won, inevitably there is a jubilant release of emotion. Sometimes we sit mesmerized watching the screen as the sports contests unfold in the conquering team. Well, the emotion in the OR is no different. It's what each of us had trained years for—in my case 11 years. The more senior MDs had trained for many more. Death had been defeated—at least at that moment—and emotion flowed.

We still needed to close the chest—a process that can take over an hour. Sutures, and sometimes small wires, are used to steadily bring tissue layers together that were intact only hours before—tissue layers that, in this case, could withstand the pounding of top-tier football tackles.

A tube was inserted into the chest cavity through a separate incision between another two ribs to re-expand the lung that collapses on the side of the chest that is open. This process is somewhat routine and does not take the concentration and focus prior events demanded. Music came on—loud music. It's not unusual to see singing and dancing around the OR table at times as people professionally and competently complete their work.

Alone as we were, unknown to the world, I can only remember that feeling (that thousands of subsequent procedures have had for me) of pure joy. Was I tired? You bet I was. Was I spent? You can count on that in the wee hours of the morning. This, however, is what I—and we as a team—was made for. How often do humans have the blissful inner glow of those feelings?

The dedication of this book may make much more sense, as you now have entered my world and my heart. To me, this is love with legs—a team of people who have trained almost unbearably intensely for years to be ready at a moment's notice to go to war for those unable to help themselves. Not everyone would feel this way. However, because I do, I know it's what I was made to do.

The mood was immediately shattered several minutes later. A barrage of out-of-character profanity from the head of the table snapped all our faces to attention.

Anesthesia care in situations like these is beyond chaotic. A physician specializing in the craft deals with pain, vacillating consciousness, blood pressure swings, blood loss, physiologic alterations as body cavities are opened and closed, nerves cut or irritated by surgical contact fire, uncontrolled bursts that can knock the airplane of human life out of the air. It's hard, on-the-edge work. To do that work in this state of controlled chaos and panic is, to me, amazingly admirable.

After interpreting changes in status in moment-to-moment decisions, multiple medications have to be drawn up and given to the patient directly into the bloodstream at the correct time in the correct dosages. In normal situations, these syringes filled with medications are clearly labeled and organized on tables at the head of the bed. In urgent trauma cases, you simply grab the vial of origin and GO, doing the best you can due to the rapid-fire events. One doesn't have the time to neatly label things. It would be as out of place as tidying up the living room before you left a burning house.

The anesthesiologist at the head of the table was one I would want working on me if I were on the table. He was one of the best in these situations I had ever seen, but in this instance, he made a terrible mistake. He had administered either a medication or a dosage of medication that was having the opposite effect on the blood pressure that we wanted. Once it is given, it can't be taken back.

The music went away, talking stopped, and the entire room watched the monitors as the effect took full hold. Helpless, we watched this young man we'd only just thrown all our strength and effort into saving. His blood pressure and heart rate rose, the machines he was connected to beeped faster and faster, alerting us to the sudden change in his vitals. The rapidity increased and reached a dangerously high level, but rather than peaking, to our horror, it only kept rising.

Our fresh repair was being assailed by a pressure that was inching higher. Then it blew—large amounts of fresh blood filled the tube coming from the chest as the repair failed, and the majority of his blood volume left his circulatory system.

In literally seconds, we went from jubilation to the panic of urgent action. Sutures were cut, wires divided, retractors replaced, blood replacement hung and infused with a rapid infuser, blood suctioned and wiped and pushed out of the way just like a few hours ago as we re-entered the chest and placed another clamp just above the torn-out sutures.

This time, however, the extreme sudden blood loss was a much more serious offense to this man's body—a body as developed and in as good shape as any human can be. Fervently and as rapidly as possible, we worked to get his circulation going by replacing his blood volume and keeping his heart beating. Back to the ABC's…

I doubt our efforts could have been accomplished any faster in the second act of this event. However, his blood pressure, and therefore the circulation, was down for several minutes. After six minutes of no oxygen circulation, the brain starts taking irreversible damage; more time equals more damage. The remainder of the body can take much more time.

We didn't know what would occur with this man's brain in this situation, but we knew it was a dire potential outcome. Hours later, we were done for the second time, and he was transferred to the ICU for another team to take over his care.

My team had to get ready for the next day's rounds, patients, and OR, and we moved on within minutes. It was a harsh lesson of how brutal medicine can be on those who practice it.

Ironically, there is a zone where the body lives and the brain dies. Testing in the ICU showed that is what had happened. No brain function was present in an otherwise healthy body.

Four days later, I sat with his mom in the ICU as she turned off the machines that kept the body of their now brain-dead son alive.

It's hard to put all the feelings associated with that night–both at the time and afterward–into words. As a young man, I never appreciated how a person can have simultaneous feelings on all ends of the emotional spectrum. Some of them I felt and still feel are. . .

- **Joy** – after 10 years of training to experience a situation where my skills would be used and desperately needed
- **Teamwork** – the marvel of like-minded individuals who were beyond me in training and behind me, all dedicated to one human in desperate need
- **Love** – expressed in preparedness and willingness to take risks as tired, less-than-perfect humans because if not us then who?
- **Tragedy** – of the fragility of life and having a supreme result fall away so quickly
- **Sorrow and Sadness** – overpower and crushing feelings watching the parent of a child that had engendered such pride and success taken without warning
- **Brutality** – that medicine and human suffering can bring on your soul
- **Honor** – at the responsibility of being on the front lines of health care ready and available

- **Daunting Reality** – at having to be ready to work again in a few minutes after a night spent in the OR in this manner. Tedious is an understatement of what medicine can be.
- **Motivation** – to prepare for excellence to be the ultimate I can be given my opportunities and abilities because people deserve it.

7

Blink

1992

SOMETIMES LIFE IS A FIGHT, and sometimes you have to hold on to it, tenaciously, with every ounce of strength. I think the more people value life, the tighter they hold on. It's a gift, after all, one that no power on earth can replace, not with any item or any riches or anything. It's precious.

It was the fourth year and second to last year of my residency at Stanford University in Otolaryngology-Head and Neck Surgery. The days were long and seemed to only get longer the closer I got to graduation, stretched further, like taffy. And like taffy being stretched, so went my energy and attentiveness. I was working as a first responder, the person who handles situations first, a gatekeeper of sorts for his or her fellow medical staff. It had been a long workday, but there was nothing serious or worth recalling.

Around seven o'clock, I and other staff and residents—about 30 of us—piled into our department's conference room for one of our regular conference meetings. As one of our professors spoke, an electric pulse, a whining ring that rose and fell in pitch, rang throughout the room. In unplanned unison, we all glanced at our pagers (I'm dating myself a little here), which simultaneously received a STAT page.

The pagers functioned as a radio, over which crackled a voice that gave us a number. We all recognized the number to the Emergency Room. It was my pager going off announcing unplanned duties that were waiting for my attention. My pulse started off, faster now, as I'm sure that of the other staff did too. STAT pages are serious. Especially when the entire staff gets it. After hustling for about a thousand yards, I reached the ER. Ducking into the hubbub of nurses, doctors, and other medical staff moving, talking, gesturing, and attending to patients, I peeked into the trauma room. The hubbub was more intense there. A sickly, sweet smell pervaded–blood, I thought, and lots of it. I looked down and saw the dark red stuff pooling on the previously clean, white floor. And whether it was subtleties in the staff's body language or just some sixth sense I had developed over four years in residency, I gathered there was an added anxiety. The tension was as pungent as the blood.

Assuming the situation the STAT call had alerted us to was there in that room, I entered. In the center of the staff's huddle was a man, somewhere in his late 20s or early 30s, lying on a gurney. He lay still, save his eyes, which blinked in panicked rapidity. It was locked-in syndrome.

Locked-in syndrome happens when a stroke occurs in a small section of the brain, which kills the neural connections within the tissue of that region. Those neural connections control physical function. When they go down, all victims can do is blink; they can't move, can't swallow, can't speak, can't even turn their head–the only movement possible is to move the eyes (only up and down and not side to side) or blink the eyelids. He had suffered in this condition for several years and was housed in a facility that could deal with his needs for complete care. He could do nothing for himself.

None of us would dispute that's a difficult life. No, it's beyond difficult. First, you're in constant discomfort—there's a catheter in your bladder and a tube that pushes food caught between a solid and a liquid form into your stomach. Your neck, specifically your trachea, has a hole surgically created in it, and into that permanent fixture, doctors place a tracheostomy tube that pumps air in and out of your lungs, a rubber windpipe with a ventilator attached. This apparatus is probably the most intrusive yet crucial to sustaining life with this extremely rare condition.

Because someone with locked-in syndrome can't cough, the tube helps suck out mucus buildup in the lungs that coughing would normally remove. On the tube's other end—inside the windpipe (medically known as the trachea), the one near the hole—is a balloon. It keeps mucus and other drainage from his salivary glands, nose, and sinuses, from filling his lungs down the trachea.

If they got down in there, he'd soon develop pneumonia. That balloon was crucial to keep him alive. Here, a foreign object—a tracheostomy tube—kept his body going, kept this incredible, organic engine from breaking down, for years now, too. And for those years, the balloon was perhaps overinflated. Remember tightening string around your finger and how if you pulled it tight enough, your finger would go numb? That's because the pressure cuts off blood flow. If the dam holds, tissues that aren't receiving blood die—necrosis is the official medical term.

In this patient's case, the balloon in his windpipe had caused tissue around it to die slowly. The subsequent necrosis ate away at the tissues surrounding and lining his innominate artery, the first branch from the aortic arch that carries blood away from the heart. Nurses at his care facility spotted blood spurting out of his trachea. Unsure of how to fix the problem, and unaware of its severity, they simply inflated the balloon. They did it a couple of times, furthering tissue damage but reducing the bleeding. After their efforts failed to remedy the problem, they brought him into the ER.

When the first-line ER doctors removed the balloon in an attempted diagnosis, the flow of blood went from a trickling brook to a raging river.

This is where I came in. As a resident specializing in head and neck surgery, I was naturally called to aid the patient. By the time I arrived, they had reflated the balloon, temporarily stemming the blood loss.

The visual record of what had transpired was grim. Those present had blood-stained uniforms; their scrubs and white coats, now partially drenched in it, had turned a deep maroon hue. When I got closer, I saw it had spattered on the curtain too. It almost felt like a scene out of a movie. I realize now it didn't faze us—we had become used to scenes that would have been extremely hard to endure before the formal process of surgical training.

The other staff rushed around, IVs in hand, to replenish the blood he'd lost. It wasn't a long-term fix by any means, but it temporarily stabilized his blood pressure by keeping the space inside his blood vessels filled, allowing the heart to circulate the life-sustaining red blood cells as they delivered oxygen to his tissues. We have a bit of margin as humans here, as we can lose over half of the red blood cells and still adequately deliver oxygen to the tissues to sustain life—if the volume lost is replaced with a saline solution of the same concentration as blood. All the while, other staff constantly battled for control of his trachea, refilling the balloon, which was struggling to hold air. If it went flat, he'd have less than two minutes.

Our chief concern turned to shuttling him into the OR—his only chance of surviving this event. There, we could repair the fistula—the opening between the artery and the trachea—and the artery. As a surgeon, that was my area of expertise, along with several other surgeons on our team.

I sometimes catch myself whining and complaining about little things: bad cell reception, traffic, even the weather. I used to do so without noticing. And I didn't see how petty those matters were until I encountered that young man with locked-in syndrome.

This was a human who, for years, had lived in a difficult state, with what I would have at one point deemed the lowest quality of life possible. He couldn't speak, couldn't respond, couldn't move or utter a sound, not even a moan; he couldn't even hug or shake hands. Still, he was a human with all the emotions, dreams, and needs as everyone else.

Before we carted him into the operation room, I wanted to check him, make sure he was still hanging with us, as he'd lost a vast amount of blood. I needed to communicate with him. As the patient, he needed to know what was happening, had the right to know and choose. I called his name and explained I understood his condition. I wasn't sure he could understand me. I realized, with full gravity of the situation, that he might not want to continue living. What if he didn't, and we saved his life—just to allow him to endure more of what must be a challenging existence?

"I'm going to ask you a series of questions to see if you're understanding me and hearing me," I told him. "I want you to blink once for yes and two for no."

He stared back at me, locking his eyes on my face. "Can you hear me?" He blinked. My heart leaped. It didn't surprise me as much as it relieved me in the center of the controlled chaos of this emergency treatment room. If he could coherently communicate, there was a chance he'd pull through. "Do you know we're at Stanford University Hospital?" was my next inquiry. Another blink. Although I was confident his responses were genuine, I had to make sure.

"Is your name ___," I asked, choosing a name that wasn't his. He blinked twice. Now that I had established a bridge for further messages, I could fully explain his options. After a few minutes of more questions, I filled him in on his situation.

"You have two choices right now. Your first option is to let us take you into the OR and fix this. It'll most likely save your life, and we can return you to the care facility afterward." I continued. "Your second option is to not enter the OR. What is going on now will take your life if we do not do anything in the next few minutes."

Before he responded, I paused. A torrent of thoughts stormed forth, arresting my momentary attention: "Would I want to live, to keep living, if my life was like this? Would I want to keep undergoing pain, enduring the life of apparatuses and machines and the tubes and the needles and the discomfort? Would it be better just to die, to just go back, and go to sleep in a comfortable bed for one final time?" Would you?

The thoughts ceased. I was still there, standing by him. I looked down at my shoes, now stained in the sweet-smelling, sticky blood that had pooled up.

I asked him if he wanted to go forward with the surgery (one blink) or not (two blinks) after giving him the time and respect to make his own choice. He blinked. I asked him again to confirm. He blinked once again. I asked a third time in a different way just to be 100% sure, apologizing but explaining I needed to be sure. He blinked yes to the new line of questioning, no to the second option; those blinks were determined, deliberate, wholeheartedly mustered. He wanted to live. As strongly as he could tell me with his small communication method, he wanted to live.

We moved to honor his wish. Only now, the bleeding had picked up. Concern started creeping in. I wasn't sure how much he'd lost, but it was a lot, and it was picking up again. I acted.

I pushed the pinky of my latex clad hand into the hole in his trachea and wedged my finger in between the balloon where the fissure in the artery had opened. Another care doctor then deflated the balloon, removed the tracheostomy tube, and inserted a fresh one with a larger higher-pressure balloon. As they inflated it, I removed my pinky. We lost some blood in the process, but it kept him alive long enough to operate on him.

A few days later, he'd recovered. My communication was still limited, and there was no ability for him to relay any emotion. Before he left the hospital, I asked him if he was happy with the decision he had made to live—one blink … yes.

8

Six Shooters

1998

MYANMAR IS A HOT, HUMID PLACE, covered in rich swathes of dense jungle. Scattered rivers, forking like veins through the vast foliage, serve as the life source of countless natives who fish and trade along their banks. Deeply rooted behind the richness of the jungle is a tangle of human rights abuses and support of the illicit drug trade. Most Americans know the country as Burma—the United States government at the time referred to the tiny nation as the "axis of evil."

I was living in a reality far away from Burma, in more ways than one. At the time, I was in my mid-30s, a few short years away from finishing my residency at Stanford University and launching into a promising medical career. So when I received a formal invitation from the Burmese government to perform surgery and teach their local surgeons my techniques—the same government so recently labeled "evil"—I was torn.

As a lifelong lover of adventure and calculated challenge, I was thrilled at the prospect of using my skills to positively impact the lives of those with no access to quality medical care. Medicine in foreign lands had always had a curious draw on my heart, and this was my first opportunity to use my skills abroad. I had nearly a decade of grueling medical training behind me and was fully confident in my skills, but I also toted a decade's worth of debt from my tuition fees. As a husband and father of three small children, I was keenly aware of the weighty consequences for my family if any harm came to me overseas. My wife, though supportive, gently reminded me of this on more occasions than one. I was deeply conflicted.

There was one major deciding factor yet to be addressed. Given the political situation in Burma, the United States required governmental permission for any American citizen to travel there. My probing request unfurled into a month-long process of interviews and questioning, involving both the Department of State and the CIA, each of which repeatedly advised against my entry into Burma. Ultimately, I was granted permission to go but on one exceedingly clear and sobering condition: I was entirely on my own. If things went wrong—whatever "wrong" entailed—there would be no intervention on my behalf. If I went to Burma, I went alone. There was no lifeline and no escape route.

But my mind was made up. I was going to go.

For me, the decision wasn't the product of mere youthful impulsiveness or naïveté. I was aware of the risks, and they weren't insignificant. But medicine had always been, for me, far more than a profession—it was my God-ordained calling, one I did not have the right to refuse. Using my skills to bring hearing to the needy in Burma wasn't just a convenient opportunity to do what I loved; it seemed a clear gateway into the career of restoration and healing I had been compelled to pursue. I was keenly aware that one day I would be called to account for the way I stewarded my gifts. I had no intention of being found wanting.

And so, a few short weeks later, I watched quietly as the twisted jungle and its flowing veins shivered into view through the thick fog beneath my descending airplane's wheels.

Military escorts met our team of three surgeons as soon as we stepped foot on the tarmac. We were immediately whisked past customs and taken directly to the US Embassy, where we completed the customary questioning, watched by hard-faced soldiers wearing guns. An assortment of local TV network and news channel employees trailed behind us everywhere we went, armed with an assortment of cameras and media paraphernalia. Their constant presence throughout the trip provided a strange comfort, a familiar cohort of followers amid the weapon-laden government troops that escorted us quite literally everywhere.

Despite the political tension, we were treated remarkably well. The local media and public relations teams heavily praised our work, and, accordingly, their viewers and the people of Burma at large did too. We had, after all, been invited to expand medical opportunities for impoverished citizens and to provide training for local physicians. It only made sense that we would be treated well. Still, this was my first exposure to a military state. It was, at least at first, somewhat unsettling. In retrospect, giving a group of foreigners a personal cohort of armed guards was actually a kind move from their government. They obviously took our well-being seriously. The assault rifles strapped to the chests of our accompaniment proved it.

During our three-week-long trip, our team of three surgeons performed surgeries in two different venues: Yangon and Mandalay. The other two surgeons focused on head and neck cancers, while I alone focused on surgery of the ear.

It's worth mentioning that all the surgeries I perform are on the microscopic level and require the use of a medical-grade microscope. I soon found out there was only one surgeon's microscope in the entire country, and it had been secured for my use. One could only hope it was in good condition.

One week into my trip, after performing approximately 20 surgeries, I again found myself seated at the operating table, peering through the lenses of this precious machine. Attached to the microscope was a camera that projected what I was seeing through the scope onto the quivering and blinking screen of a tiny 10-inch monitor.

Around the screen huddled a crowd of local ear, nose, and throat doctors. There were 27 of them per my recollection, virtually all the ENT physicians in the country. All of them were there to observe me as I operated on a patient with severe hearing loss caused by a condition known as otosclerosis.

Normally, sound that strikes the eardrum is transmitted through the ear by means of three tiny middle ear bones, also known as ossicles, into the inner ear and onward to the brain. Otosclerosis is characterized by the abnormal formation of bony scar tissue around the third bone of hearing, a stirrup-shaped bone known as the stapes. This causes the stapes to become fused and immobile, severely limiting the vibrations it normally passes on to the inner ear and brain.

The surgical treatment for this condition is to remove a portion of the stapes and drill a tiny opening through the base of the bone that extends into the fluid-filled inner ear. And by tiny, I mean just that—tiny. The opening I needed to make was 0.8 millimeters in diameter. At home, we typically used a precise laser to make the hole. A physician who had previously worked at my practice had invented the laser. In this part of the world, there would be no way to access that technology. We would have to do it the old-fashioned way, manually, with a drill and a submillimeter margin of error.

After drilling the hole, the portion of the stapes that had been removed would need to be replaced with a prosthesis, with one end connected to the remaining middle ear bones and the other end delicately inserted into the tiny hole. In this way, a mobile chain for sound conduction would be restored; sound vibrations contacting the eardrum would then be transmitted through the mobile prosthesis into the inner ear as they should be. In short, if all went according to plan, this patient's hearing could be successfully and completely restored.

(If this is difficult to understand, you can visit http://www.californiaearinstitute.com/surgical-services-laser-stapedotomy-video.php for a more detailed explanation.)

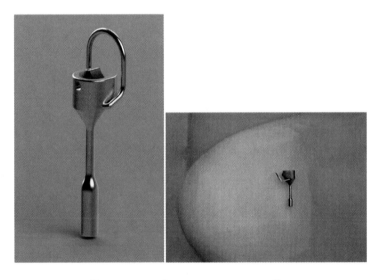

Stapes prostheses are very small,
measuring 4 mm long x 0.6 mm at the tip

Lacking chairs, all 27 of the local physicians sat on the dirt floor, peering expectantly at the monitor. The heat hung heavy and low, pressed thickly against our faces by the extreme humidity. The only window in the room was propped open, an invitation for all things that fly to enter.

I sat, as relaxed as one could be with dime-sized drops of sweat rolling down his back, and with 27 expectant spectators.

In the states, I would do this procedure in an OR brought up to the standards of medicine in the 21st century, outfitted with top-tier medical technology afforded by the American medical industry. The patient would be adequately sedated, but not under full general anesthesia, as was the case here. But this was Myanmar, and my 20-year-old female patient did not speak English. To keep the language barrier from confusing things further, I agreed to let the local Burmese anesthesiologist put the patient completely to sleep.

As he busied himself putting the proper sedatives into the patient's IV, I began to explain the functions of the equipment I had brought with me to the local physicians. My "ear set" of OR tools contains 179 small instruments equipped with various curves, edges, and configurations to perform specific functions deep within a patient's skull base.

The Burmese "ear set" the government courteously offered me contained a total of 6 instruments. I had courteously declined, explaining that I had brought my own tools. As I withdrew each instrument from the kit, each was met with wide-eyed stares and hushed murmurs of amazement. These tools were the work of hundreds of surgeons over the years. Without them, I could not come close to executing many of the delicate procedures I regularly perform.

Each surgeon compiles his or her own personal instrument set over the course of their training and career; mine was a product of years of training and practice. I had discovered many of these tools by watching the most masterful surgeons in my field, and they had proved invaluable to specific parts of each surgery I performed. I had designed and created several especially for me. The skills I had acquired, in combination with this shiny array of surgical instruments, were this patient's chance at having her hearing restored. It was time to begin.

As I lowered my hands to the job, the wide-eyed gaze of the physicians slid as one back to the monitor displaying the view from my microscope. I explained each step at length as I worked, slowly and with great caution, so that the audience might not only understand the procedure but also gain critical, first-hand understanding of what a safe and appropriately cautious surgery looked like. Normally, I would complete such a procedure in 45 minutes or less. Here, I expected to operate for 2 hours or more, for the sake of learning.

Midway through the surgery, some of my equipment began malfunctioning. It had already been hot, but now it was growing impossibly hotter. The humidity seemed to be congealing around me, the moisture-ridden air swelling with its own weight as the sun rose and the day marched on.

The doctors watched as I fiddled with the finicky gear, fighting to put it all back in working order, and sweating even harder than before. It was 30 minutes before I achieved some semblance of functionality again and bent again to the task at hand. Still ahead was the most risky, delicate stage of the surgery: the creation of the minuscule hole in the stapes (called a stapedotomy). It's an uneasy feeling having to depend on the undependable, but I had no choice.

With my faulty equipment limping along, I focused the microscope deep into the middle ear—past the eardrum that had been delicately elevated and preserved to be put back into position after the prosthesis was put in place. The movements at this stage are exceedingly intricate—so intricate, in fact, that the ability needed to properly perform them has been described as "teetering on the edge of human ability." What was my margin of error, you ask? I'll tell you—a tenth of a millimeter, at most, a hair, and a small one at that. It is easy to understand why a microscope is necessary for these procedures.

On a good day, I would be well-rested, undistracted, in a familiar setting, with the privilege of the latest high-tech and fully functional equipment. Even then, this type of surgery would require intense focus. Here, the scenario was quite different. I know I am a bit of an outlier in this, but I am happiest in the face of a challenge. The pressure of needing to do something that is just barely achievable (on a good day) is exactly where I am at my best. Little did I know the pressure that was about to present itself.

I was edging my instrument toward my millimeter's thick target when my peripherals detected a subtle but sudden shift in the room. Something was off; I didn't know what, but it was veritably tangible. The natural hum and bustling noise of the OR itself were suddenly hushed. I straightened my back, lifting my face from the eyepiece of the microscope, and surveyed the room before me.

The physicians, still seated, had previously kept up a steady stream of chatter among themselves; now they sat silent. Dead silent. And they weren't moving either. They held themselves stiffly like statues, eyes no longer on the monitor, gazes locked fearfully on the floor, seemingly doing their best to disappear altogether. It was like one of those scenes in an old pioneer movie, when the forest, with all its birds, frogs, and any other critters, slips into a pregnant silence just before the Indians or whatever unseen foe attacks. I scanned the scene repeatedly, trying to make sense of whatever had raised the hairs on the back of my neck.

Then, I heard it. Somewhere, down some passage and in some other room of the hospital, was a jingling sound, like keys on a key chain. At first, it was faint and remote, barely enough to register; but as I listened it grew louder, louder—and closer. It was approaching our room, escalating in volume as it came. At last, it was almost on top of us, and right as it reached peak volume … it ceased altogether. The sound had stopped directly behind me. Steadying my nerves, I spun collectedly to face whoever or whatever was there.

Before me stood five stolid feet of Myanmar's military elite. The short, stout figure appeared to be that of a high-ranking commander—a Napoleon of a man, chin held high. His chest glistened with rows on rows of medals—the source of the jingling. His jacket, which bore them, hung heavy under the weight of his accolades and strained around an abundant gut.

Strapped to the wide belt around his waist was a pair of shining, pearl-handled revolvers—a six-shooter for each hand. The bulldog expression on his face exuded a threatening flatness. His was a face accustomed to unquestioned authority, and his expression made it clear that this encounter would be no exception. His eyes locked onto mine, icy and menacing. I was neither too foolish nor too courageous to let my eyes wander from his. I managed to smile politely.

"How's it going?" The little conqueror inquired. The room remained utterly silent, the heads of my audience still bowed fearfully. There was a pause as I scrambled for what to say. I had a strong suspicion my first impression would matter with this fellow.

"It's going well, sir. Thank you," I responded. The next move would be his.

He stared me down. Silence. It felt even hotter now. And more humid too.

"Do you know who that is?" he asked, nodding abruptly to the patient lying sedated on the operating table.

I was mightily tempted to lie in that moment. GUESS, my brain hissed. It was a reactionary panic, a primal urge to feign confidence. I did not know who this man was, but, judging from the body language of those around us, he was a source of extreme respect or terror or, more likely, both. I was an American citizen in a country whose government didn't exactly see eye to eye with my own—and we had labeled them the "axis of evil." Whoever he was, I knew with complete certainty that I wanted to stay in good graces with him and faking it would not make it here. I fought the urge, reclaimed my judgment, and answered honestly, "No, sir. I don't."

He said nothing again. I wondered fleetingly if my answer was the right one, or, if not, what on earth would have been. His little hands came to rest on the grips of his twin pistols.

Finally, he looked back at me. "That," he gestured grandiosely at the woman on the table, "is my wife."

Another pause.

"I sincerely hope it goes well," he finished.

Before I could muster a response, he turned on his heel and marched out of the room. The jingling marched with him, slowly fading from earshot. No one spoke. I vaguely heard the insects that had entered the OR through the open window, buzzing aimlessly about. For the first time that day, I didn't mind the sound.

It felt as though gravity had taken a special interest in me and left everything but the speck of earth I occupied untouched. That little man had clearly illuminated how serious my situation was. I myself had seen bullet wounds in the trauma bay; I had seen the damage they could do. I was personally acquainted with life and death. This surgery needed to be a success, or it seemed clear that I would get to know them on even more intimate terms.

Suspended over the flames of the little general's threats, I leaned heavily on my mantle of experience and training as a surgeon. My mind raced. Leaving was no option, and neither was failure. I could just wait for my patient to wake up and tell her we'd run into difficulty and had to abort surgery. I could even blame my equipment;

it had, after all, been faulty, and any reasonable person would understand that ... right? But maybe this man wasn't reasonable. He had no reason to be. I was playing roulette with two six-shooters, and the only way to guarantee a blank was to get this surgery done.

My wife's words of warning—her advice to stay away from this trip, to stay home, to stay with our family—flooded back to me. The irony of potentially meeting my end over someone else's wife was not lost on me. I prayed fervently for grace.

"You're going to stay here," I told myself. "You're going to stay here, and you're going to nail this surgery with perfection. This matters. Buckle down, get to work, and do this. You have what it takes. Get it right."

I took a deep breath, looked around, and again placed my eyes to the microscope. There was no turning back.

A short time later, I was finished. The prosthesis I myself had patented lay secure and snug in its proper position; the eardrum had been delicately replaced to its original position. It could not have been done more perfectly.

Anesthesia was reversed, and the woman gradually woke up. Amazingly, the patient's hearing normally improved immediately upon placement of the prosthesis if everything went correctly. The entire room held its breath as we tested her hearing for the first time.

She was hearing.

I felt the weight roll off of me. My heart fluttered in relief, released from the burden of impending doom. I breathed a prayer of thanks and, rising to my feet, walked far away from that OR table.

After this surgery, I saw our armed escorts through a more skeptical, guarded lens. I was less trusting and less optimistic. My experience with the general awakened me afresh to my utter mortality and helplessness. It had been a sobering reminder of my incapability to save myself in the face of complete and total vulnerability.

By the grace of God, I had lived, but much of my preexisting naïveté had been put to death. I knew now this country would give me no mercy. Any discontented authority could simply wait until my back was turned, squeeze a trigger, and bury me with a convincing story—or just a bribe. Here, certain lives were valuable, and others were not. Mine was valuable only as long as I did exactly what was expected of me.

Two weeks later, my team and I sat in Yangon in a special holding area with our armed escorts, awaiting our departure flight away from the other passengers. It was a sparsely furnished room with a tiny air conditioner that was ill-suited for its job. A series of large windows looked out onto the sweltering tarmac. I turned over the events of the past few weeks in my mind. It had been an exciting and rewarding adventure, despite the near-constant worry of harm befalling my team and me. Truthfully, I had learned a staggering amount from my time in Burma. But I was ready to get home. I was tired, strained from the heat and long hours and poor diet, coupled with travelers' gastrointestinal distress.

The plane, an old DC10, roared into view. It landed uncomfortably close to the room where we sat, pulling up on the concrete of the runway with a curdling shriek, not blunted in the slightest by the walls of the waiting area. The usual armed guards ushered the other passengers aboard first and finally indicated it was our turn to go. In the absence of a proper terminal, we plunged through the door into the swirling fumes and marched across the tarmac toward the metal bird with her stairs to the ground, resting 300 yards away.

"Only 300 yards," I told myself. "300 yards are all that lies between you and your wife, your family, your country." I wasted no time in striding purposefully toward the plane's open doors. Since that fateful day in the OR, things had gone remarkably smoothly, but I knew I was not safe until I was truly safe. The sky above us stretched warmly in its expanse, not a cloud in the sky.

Only 150 yards to go. Halfway there. The muscles in my legs tensed expectantly as I drew ever nearer to the plane that would bear me far away from the tangled depths of the "axis of evil."

100 yards.

A screeching sound rent the air into a million pieces. Wheeling around, we were confronted by a glistening motorcade of military vehicles. A jet-black Jeep with large Myanmar flags streaming overhead on both sides led the charge. Between the flags glinted a roof-mounted machine gun. Two troop carriers packed full with armed soldiers sped closely behind. After them, a black limousine; behind that, two more troop-laden carrier vehicles; and another Jeep with an identical machine gun mounted in front of the furiously flapping flags.

The convoy tore down the runway, skidding to a halt in formation between us and the plane. Before I could speak or act, one of the limousine doors opened, revealing my worst fear—the general himself, six-shooters still at his hip. He was seated in the back of the limo with his wife beside him. Her eyes were fixed stolidly on the floor of the limo.

The general snapped his fingers, beckoning me to approach. He said nothing. I obeyed without hesitation, heart thudding sickly in my chest.

"How are you, Ma'am?" I managed to say to his wife. "I hope you're feeling well."

She nodded softly. As she did, the general's hand lowered toward his side. Images of the pearl-handled revolvers, of gunshot victims in the ER, of the bullet wounds I had seen up close, of my wife and kids, all flashed through my mind. I flinched inwardly. I had healed his wife, but this was Myanmar.

But rather than a blazing sidearm, out came a small box. His flat and icy gaze had not changed. He offered no smile. He shoved the box into my hands as though it were a wad of cash. "Open it," he commanded.

Inside, I found an intricately elegant oval-shaped container made of pure hammered silver. About three inches wide and five inches long, it was beautiful. I lifted my eyes to meet his one last time, and he nodded curtly. With that, the limo door was slammed shut, and they were gone. I boarded my plane, overwhelmed with relief and simple thankfulness. I would soon be with my family, in a country where I enjoyed luxuries many around the world would never know.

That little silver box now rests on a shelf beside my desk where I keep a number of small treasures, each from a different adventure. It is unassuming but, to me, it represents the journey of a lifetime, a journey from which I might never have returned from alive. On tough days, I look at it and smile inwardly and remind myself, "I have seen worse." Thankfully, I returned with a box—and not in one.

9

A Choice

1998

THE PLANE RIDE had been a long one. We'd already stopped in Bangkok, Thailand on an overnight layover and had only just hit the tarmac in Yangon, Myanmar. Twenty-seven hours of travel is fatiguing, mixed with the disparity of your internal body clock telling you it is the middle of the night and your eyes seeing midday sunshine. This was the same trip during which I had an unforgettable encounter with a man—whose name I never learned—I call the Napoleon of Myanmar. I mentioned there was a book's worth of other stories I brought home from that trip—this is one of them.

As noted previously, we were working with local surgeons, sharing our experiences with them, teaching them, and, hopefully, making them even better surgeons. We went arm in arm with soldiers who had guns, body armor, helmets, the whole shebang.

After our plane touched the tarmac, we watched through the windows as a military-looking convoy rolled onto the black asphalt and toward our airplane. One of the cabin doors opened and in came a burly, hairy soldier from the front of the airplane. His jaw was big, his arms, thick. He had no neck. "Where are the American doctors?" he thundered, with a touch of gruff authority. Not accustomed to refusals, I thought. I looked around, feeling the same nervousness I felt in my gut and that showed itself in the faces of my colleagues. After a pause, we identified ourselves, still reserved and cautious. No other passengers moved. It seemed they were glad we were the center of this man's attention.

He ordered us off the plane, accompanied by six or so other soldiers clearly under his command. After hastily gathering what luggage we had, we descended from the air-conditioned fuselage into the warm embrace of a jungle climate and were scooped up into a van, flanked by armed soldiers—none of whom appeared too happy or kindly—that lay center in the file of jeeps and armored trucks.

One moment, we were riding, and the next moment, we were ushered out of our ride into a dazzling and dizzying crowd of lights, cameras, and reporters. They had been waiting for our arrival in a marked-off corner of the airport's ground floor, in a separate building from the main terminal just to the side of the tarmac. Officials greeted us, shaking our hands, embracing us cordially. From a podium in one corner of the space, boisterous speakers vigorously delivered speeches of welcome, and thanks, and of sincere excitement at the prospect of having doctors from a country as advanced as the United States come to treat their fellow citizens. The media present, we soon learned, would accompany us our entire three-week trip.

After that, the convoy—which consisted of two jeeps in the lead, a four-wheel-drive sort of jeep-truck vehicle with a mounted machine gun, our van, and the same vehicles in reverse order behind us—whisked us from the jungle-like, rural area that surrounded the airport to Yangon. We traveled through tight, unpaved streets past traffic lights, pedestrians, and crosswalks, through a maze of ram-shackle buildings, tawdry and dilapidated. Wild dogs, beggars, all the marks of a third-world country, flew by as we moved unimpeded down roads of varying size and flatness. Our drivers, whose recklessness pushed us faster and faster through the winding lanes, took no mercy on nor notice of the many curbs we ran over nor stop-signs and red lights we ran. I was honestly afraid we were going to strike someone down in the street. There was no stopping for those drives. When facing our entourage, pedestrians had two simple choices—get out of the way or get run over.

The convoy eventually slammed to a halt at our housing, our base of operation where we'd stay during the trip—the United States embassy. Here, there were no speeches, no crowds—a concrete wall lined with razor wire, a glum wall but inside a green and beautiful courtyard full of trees and lush flowering landscaping, and more guards with helmets, body armor, and guns. Initially, going from the airport to that embassy was like leaving a game show and heading straight to an oasis. We were housed in rooms with two double beds along a long hall on the second floor. Shortly after we debarked, were pleasantly surprised by a joyous staff eager to host us and attend to our needs. Their efforts to feed us and make our stay easy were generous and well-appreciated.

The next day, I visited a local hospital to discuss our action plan and establish an itinerary for the next few days with the staff who'd be accompanying us. With the local MDs, our plan was to map out and discuss the coming surgeries. Here is where training can be tailored to the needs of the local professionals. With one-to-one interaction, it is easy to determine their level of ability or inexperience, comfort or anxiety, experience or bewilderment regarding certain procedures. Usually, it's best to pick a surgery that is not mundane to your mentees nor one that overwhelms them with something completely beyond their ability. It would be like putting a major league pitcher on the mound against a 10-year-old learning to bat—completely overwhelming and discouraging and maybe even dangerous!

Every surgeon—every good one at least—wants to meet his patients before treating them. As a general who carefully examines a map of the battlefield he's about to fight on, I read each patient's case file carefully as a substitute. Seemingly minor details can lead to success or failure, and learning these details is important for local surgeons. We have a somewhat cynical but true saying in medicine and surgery that "judgment comes from experience and experience comes from poor judgment." In short, it is the duty of surgeons further down the road to impart the lessons they have learned (sometimes through mistakes of their own) so that future patients and surgeons don't learn the same lessons again and again.

Unlike that of the United States, standard medical practice in Myanmar and many other societies don't require surgeons to discuss a procedure, risks, benefits, and other possible outcomes with a patient. Stateside, we do. It's called "informed consent."

While talking through some of the cases with the staff, one of them informed me that I would be able to select the patients to give the staff the best learning opportunity possible. As our hosts, they not only controlled our movements but our schedule.

I followed one of my scrub-clad colleagues to a pre-operating room with painted cement block walls and simple wooden furniture. There, we found seven or eight patients and their family members surrounding them, perhaps 30 people in all—all patients had life-threatening ailments. All of them were NPO (which stands for the Latin phrase *nothing per oris*), meaning they hadn't eaten or drunk anything since midnight the day before—standard for people expected to undergo anesthesia. Their heads were buzzed bald, including the women, another telling sign of their appointed operations; hair can infect a wound or incision, so we cut it around whatever area we plan to operate.

They looked at me closely, watching me as I entered this room they had been waiting in for some time. There was an air of expectancy and a wall of looming tension. I have said it before regarding work I have done in Peru, but surgery in countries as poor as Myanmar can be far more dangerous; medical science hasn't advanced far there yet.

No one spoke. The would-be patients stood, looking at me still. As I looked back at them, the local staff told me there was only time for three operations. Here was twice, almost three times that many people. Each case was presented to me—x-rays, hearing tests, lab tests, physical findings, and details …

"I thought we were only operating on three?" I asked one of my hosts. "That's right," he responded, arms crossed, looking about, scanning the room. "Choose your three patients from these."

Here were people, dear people, all with lives, families, people they loved, all with life-threatening ailments, and still, they didn't fuss, or cry out, or anxiously plead. The dignity and the indignity of the situation struck me like a blast furnace.

The dangerous reality of their plight was simple—each had some sort of tumor, infection, or deadly malady. An operation was their best shot at survival. There in that evaluation room near the OR, they waited patiently, trustingly even, for treatment, their lives hanging precariously in the balance. Their heads shaved and bellies emptied, all had entered that pre-operating room hoping they would go into surgery and walk out to live their life with their family.

Waking in my embassy room earlier that day, I had been filled with a wondrous sense of optimism at the prospects of helping people, at the work we'd be doing, at the aid we'd be bringing, and the people whose lives we'd better. Now I held that terrible, sovereign scepter of choice. I had already reviewed each patient's case history. I looked at each of them, at their eyes.

"What if this were me?" I asked myself. "Or worse, what if one of these people were my child, my wife, a parent, or a sibling?" My mind started racing; who gets priority? And why? How do I choose? Should it be those most in pain or those who could least afford an operation?

I felt I would be leaving the four or five I couldn't operate on to die. I felt terrible. I could feel my stomach swirling, my breakfast, some mortar of dread and guilt. The flood of questions passed quickly though, and, despite my grievance, I made a decision. Quickly too.

"We're doing all the cases," I said.

"Not possible," the local staff retorted.

"Then we do none of them," I shot back.

I wouldn't budge. As the chief surgeon, I swept aside their refusals with that scepter of authority, and two days later–two days of long hours, of little sleep, of fatigue and weariness–I finished surgery on all the patients. I can promise you their medical staff will never forget those 48 hours, and neither will I.

The experience opened my eyes to the thousands of people, millions even, out in the world, not just Myanmar, who are in desperate need of medical care. It really centered me, a young physician who'd only just begun his career, and made me reckon and grapple with a question every surgeon faces: What is my responsibility and how do I balance need with what's realistic? As a follower of Jesus, it imposed a similar, more specific question I still ask myself: How do I share the blessing of medical care and shoulder other demands and responsibilities? I don't see a time when Jesus refused a person in a medical need. That's a high bar.

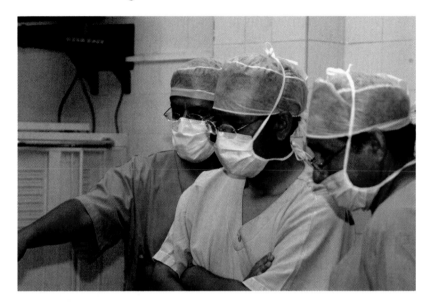

As a younger surgeon, sometimes my gut instinct to help overrode all other judgment. It certainly did in that hospital in Yangon, Myanmar. Every one of those 48 hours, difficult as they were, undoubtedly were worth it. Afterward, I slept deep and peacefully, and harder than I had in months. I don't think I could have if I hadn't made such a choice. I think my sleep would still be disturbed by the eyes of those who had been left to die if I had not made that decision many years ago in a country far away.

10

Only a Man

2002

TWO DAYS–Monday and Tuesday specifically–that's how long it took my team to perform 10 cochlear implants.

The year was 2004, and I found myself in Lima, Peru with one of our Let Them Hear Foundation teams performing implants and teaching well-respected, local physicians to do the same–fishing and teaching others to as well.

Each surgery, each success made a world of difference for each child. The ten we'd worked on rested together after their procedures had been completed, each marked with our trademark purple bandage. That was Monday and Tuesday. Later in the week, we'd test out the implants and tune them to ensure they were functioning properly.

Meanwhile, their families–waiting with eager anticipation–bristled with excitement, overwhelmed with joy at the prospect their children would soon possess the gift of hearing.

At this point on most of our trips, I'm pretty mentally wired. Having spent a day or two in the high-strung tension of an OR–a zone we call the "redline"–I'm generally energetic come evening (or whenever I finally step away from work-related tasks). This trip was no exception.

I stood on our hotel room's balcony looking out over the dusty, urban sea that is Lima. There, seated over a chunk of Peruvian society and culture, over a city gurgling with sound and smells and sights and just life in general, my mind turned to the events of days before, to the surgeries and the patients, the possible outcomes, the possibilities. I mulled over each surgery, each point of learning my physician-trainees had received. I had let one of them perform the surgery, step-by-step, himself; I had only accompanied him as a guide. I fixated on that trainee. *Can he do it? I mean the surgery. Can he really do it? By himself, too?*

My thoughts cycled further on.

And what were our objectives when we started this trip? Were we accomplishing them? And whether yes or no, what would come next?

I started down my mental checklist of answers, totally enraptured in my introspection, like someone overcome by the heavy air of some intoxicating odor.

Then, like the slow, creeping tide, the realization of how privileged I was to do this—these surgeries for children, all over the world, to work in this field, to have had the opportunity to become a surgeon, and to share the love of Christ in the way He'd created me to—rolled over me.

This revelation pushed me to look deeper, not at the events of days past, but at a broader picture. In the enveloping twilight that had begun to slowly drape the city below, I turned my mind's eye to our operations and the heart behind what we do.

I thought about eight months ago when we first announced that we'd be seeking children who needed implants. I had developed several dozen criteria for our team to select candidates and rank patients from first to last in order of importance. Our goal was to give the highest chance of success in the procedure to prove to the locals that this does, in fact, work. Things like age (younger is better), normal anatomy (we need a place to place the delicate electrode in the inner ear so it can stimulate the hearing system), supportive family, etc. have all been shown to increase the chance of outstanding outcomes.

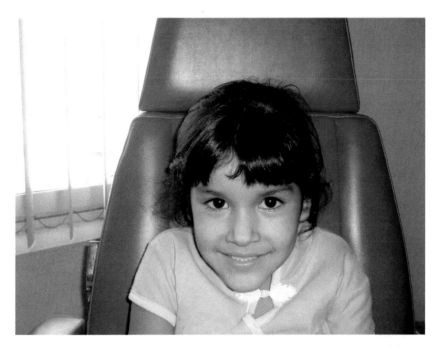

It's hard to face choices like this objectively. A heap of social and cultural factors influences this sort of decision-making. Saying yes to some and no to others is a brutally emotional process. We reject candidates—children who need help—knowing they'll suffer from the difficulties of deafness for the rest of their lives. Many of them are caught in rather desperate situations. For example, one boy we treated in Peru (there's a video about him at www.LetThemHear.org) was suffering from a condition that not only caused progressive deafness but blindness too. His father had taken a job working construction—his second job at that point—to pay off the hearing aid he'd purchased his son but had died in an accident on the job.

Fortunately, we were able to treat him, but, sadly, many like him will never receive the proper care they need.

As my thoughts ran on, I felt two streams of emotion surface in my heart. The first was extreme joy and gratitude at the prospect and the opportunity to change ten lives in the city I now watched from my perch; for the generous donors whose contributions made it possible; for a hardworking team; for the willingness of the local MD who'd be running the clinic here; for the 12 years of schooling and training that had prepared me for this work; for the fact I was born in a country where I had the opportunity to tune and develop my skills as both a physician and teacher; and for a supportive family, without whom this would never have happened.

The second stream was one of sorrow. At least 200 children (maybe more) who'd applied were turned down. Although it took a herculean effort to do just those ten, when I tore away all my other sentiments, all other factors, until I was left with a purely subjective standpoint, I realized our work barely scratched the surface of the overall need we faced in Lima. And this wouldn't be the only case in which we'd have to forgo treating a large majority of those in need. It's the reality of this field of work, an inescapable one—at least if you're being realistic and honest with yourself.

As the city bathed in moonlight and quietly throbbed with evening life, I was overcome with a hurricane of emotion, overcome by the feelings of gratitude and despair at what seemed to be utter hopelessness. I wept.

I think many medical professionals feel these emotions. They build up, like methane gasses underground, and sometimes, like that night in Lima, they burst forth and catch you like a gut punch.

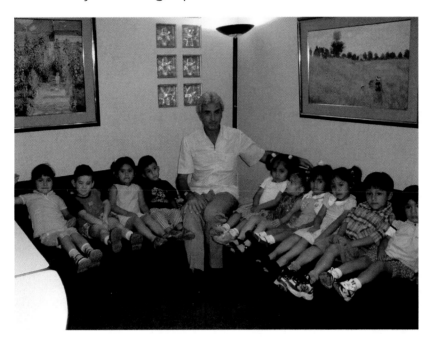

There have only been a few times I felt my Maker's presence like I did in those next few moments. I couldn't hear anything—at least like you'd hear someone talking to you face to face—or see a form or being or some light, but there was a presence I could feel.

There was communication; I felt words coming forth. I can't really articulate it, because it's something you have to experience to fully understand it. Regardless, I felt peace overcome me. It sliced through the pain and complexity of the situation. I knew God knew what I felt; He knew my anguish, and He knew this tension of gratitude and despair I found myself in.

Not through audible words or vivid pictures, but some humanly impossible means of communication, God transmitted words into my mind.

"You are only a man," came first.

"A bit brutal," I thought.

He continued: "I am so pleased with you for doing what you can. I am so pleased with you for seeing My people's needs and responding. That's the best and all you can do in your life."

The warmth in my heart is beyond comparison; again, human articulation is inadequate.

It proceeded again: "What you need is someone to be able to speak a word and change this place in an instant, in a permanent way. You will never be able to fix this yourself. I am your ultimate hope and nothing else."

And that was it; it was over, and the words ceased. But those words of comforting guidance I felt so strongly impressed upon my soul while sitting above Lima, Peru, brought lasting freedom into my life. Afterward, I lived with the understanding that I was to address the needs presented to me without feeling I had to fix it all, unchained from the despair and feelings of inadequacy.

As humbling as it is, it's a pleasant comfort for me to know and say, "I'm only a man."

11

I Know Why You Came

2007

CHOOSING WHERE TO TRAVEL for a new Let Them Hear Foundation trip is a daunting task. The need in our world is immense, and the desire to maximize the treasure others give us to do this work is a primary motivator. We also want to achieve a lasting influence and site so that more than just those children we treat benefit, which starts with our arrival. We want a functioning, good team to carry on the work we do in the beginning.

The need is absolutely massive. If all the children born with hearing loss in the world over the next ten years grew to adulthood and then joined hands, how far do you think it would reach? If it started in California where I live and went east, would it go to the Sierras? The Rockies? The Mississippi River? Actually, it would reach 2.5 times around the earth! Ninety-five percent of those children will be born to families that have no history of deafness. No matter where we go, our efforts are not even a scratch on the surface of this massive human health issue.

We take the decision on where to go seriously and bathe it in hard, objective criteria for selection, but there's also an intangible factor—prayer. It's a sort of "East meets

West" conflict when picking a destination. I am comparing the decision to the hyper-data-based medicine of the Western world and the sometimes mystical, non-scientific medicine of some parts of the developing world. We can get data that provides the number of cochlear implant centers per population and estimates of the number of children born deaf, physicians available for training, the difficulty of visas and travel documents, etc.

With prayer, the answers are more subtle and usually less concrete. Sometimes it's a door that opens, sometimes a sequence of events showing the way, sometimes only a subjective feeling of non-verbal communication. Even after we have decided and all the way through the actual trip, I always have in the back of my mind the question, "Was this the place we were supposed to go?"

Our team of medical professionals (including an MD surgeon, nurses, audiologists, OR scrub nurses, etc.) traveled to a tiny village deep in the mountains of China. The heart of Americans to go and do and help has been incredibly encouraging over the years, and on this trip, we had 20+ others with us.

Our group frequently performs acts of kindness for those in need. We have seen individuals equip entire orphanages with mattresses, fund education for children, adopt children—the list is long and joyous. Not unlike other villages in the mostly agrarian, communist nation, men farm, selling the food they harvest to feed their own families. Electricity is absent, as are motorized vehicles. For residents there, seeing one would be as foreign as a horse and buggy to a New Yorker.

And in that village lived Li Bing. He was nine when we first met. He was a quiet boy, deaf—though not from birth. His family was clothed in the fine, ceremonial dress of the mountain tribes of Western China. Brightly colored and exquisite in quality, their fashion spoke of the seriousness of this day in their lives. It was his father who would provoke me with a seemingly simple comment. The man was small, muscular, the product of a hard life of farming, of scraping up just enough resources for his family and himself.

I had traveled thousands, tens of thousands of miles before then, and from the United States to South America to Asia, and everywhere else in between, no one had asked me that question. Before now at least. I looked at him and his wife, and their son. I looked at my translator and back at him.

Although the little boy was one of many, we'd be treating on one of our LTHF trips to China, his mother and father felt their boy would be treated with distinct honor, hence the ornate garb. Over the bridge of language our translator created, manned, and held for the duration of the trip, I conversed with his parents. In humble excitement, they shared Li Bing's story.

As a young child, Li Bing fell hard into a dangerous illness. Remote and poor, the village lacked any establishment of medicine. One evening, after a few days of battling the dangerously high temperature, Li Bing collapsed into unconsciousness. His father bore him in his arms, carrying him for nine hours until he reached the nearest clinic.

It must have been agony to burden and strain under the weight of a sick child through the night; I can attest to that as a parent. It kills you to watch your children suffer, and here was a boy who, for days, had been ravaged by fever and had now fallen into what his father may have believed was fatal. I wonder what it must have been like to walk holding an unresponsive child for so long on such a lonely journey.

He'd reached the clinic just after daybreak. The boy was still alive. Doctors quickly supplied him an IV and stabilized his vitals. Two weeks later, he returned to his village with his father. Although the wave of symptoms had abated, the bacterial infection and illness, having gone untreated for quite a time, had taken its toll; doctors diagnosed the boy with meningitis, Li Bing's father told me.

For some time, his cerebrospinal fluid—the fluid that fills the inner ear through a tiny duct in the skull's base bone—had fallen under attack from the meningitis, effectively damaging his nervous system, and even the brain itself. Whether the infection started near the brain and spread to the inner ear or vice versa, I'm unsure—either is possible. Regardless, with the same ruthlessness of a Weedwacker being used on a bed of flowers, the infection had killed the sensitive and delicate nerve endings that normally rest in the shelter of the cochlea, an organ of the inner ear.

Fortunately, patients suffering from deafness by meningitis, like Li Bing, make ideal cochlear implant candidates. Despite the damage his inner ear nerve endings sustained, the infection hadn't touched the nerve that carries the signal from them into the brain. Li Bing's inner ear nerve endings were also fully developed. And that wasn't all working in his favor. In some meningitis cases, the patient's ear forms a bone in the cochlea as a reaction to the infection; it's difficult to remove but necessary if we're to perform an implant since it blocks off the exact area where the implant would go. We were relieved upon discovering its absence in a CT scan—a special sort of x-ray.

Via our faithful translator (a good translator is worth more than their weight in gold abroad), I explained the surgery, the entire process, including recovery times, risks, and possible outcomes, with Li Bing's father and mother. They loved that boy with a pure intensity evident to all. I didn't need to know their language to tell that. In fact, I have seen that everywhere I have traveled. It's a tangible, universal sentiment that one catches in nonverbal cues and facial expressions.

I think it eludes sight or sound (vocal inflection). It's innate, instinctual; you sniff it out with experience, and the more you are confronted with it, the more you know it. I think that's because it appeals to something in all of us— the willingness to sacrifice oneself for another we love dearly, the thing we count most precious. Our children are indeed in that category. And I'm sure China's "one-child policy" made the whole situation all the more desperate—and the love Li Bing's parents had for him—only more apparent.

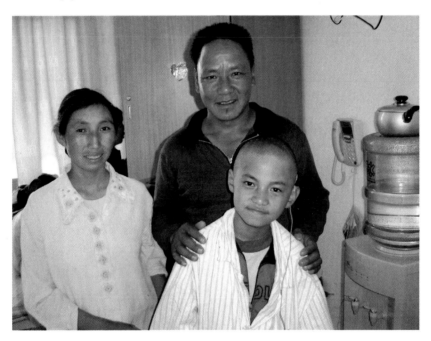

After I finished the lecture, Li Bing's father said something to the translator, who turned to me and asked, "This sounds expensive, why do you do it?" I felt honored (and always do with this question), explaining how I had experience and could help people, why I wanted to help people with my special skills, and why people in the USA believed in such a mission and had donated their money to see it carried out. I wasn't sure he'd understand.

He listened and turned to the translator again. "I would like to help with the cost. I have a cow, two chickens, and a pig," he said. "You can have the pig and the chickens to help pay for it. I cannot give you the cow, or my family could not survive the winter." I was stunned. My heart was moved in a way it had never been. After that, I think I better understood why Li Bing's parents had dressed in the finest garb they had for the boy.

The surgery went smoothly—no hiccups and no snags. So did the programming. It's a tedious process that happens about four or five days after the surgery and involves tuning each of the 23 electrodes in the implant. We run an electric current through each one, slowly increasing it until it stimulates the electrode and transfers the signal to the brain, which interprets it as sound—success, or in doctor's terms, reaching the threshold or "T level." We then work it up to the highest level the patient can withstand "C level"—the comfort level.

By the way, sound gets progressively louder from the threshold T-level to the maximum comfortable C-level. This effectively determines the working range of current for programming. After the individual electrodes are tuned, we turn them all on simultaneously. It takes about an hour or two—longer in the case of a language barrier.

When it came time for tuning, both Li Bing's parents (they had been there for the whole thing) and I intently observed the audiologist. Audiologists, not surgeons, fit hearing aids and run the electrode tests, including programming the cochlear implants. I had seen them do their work plenty of times, and the technical aspect was impressive.

But that's not what I noticed, not what was glaring, drawing my attention forth. No, it was Li Bing's parent's, their seriousness. They had waited, watched the entire time, silent, still as stone statues. They were fixated upon the scene. War could have broken out in the hills around the village, and they still would have watched on, watched their son.

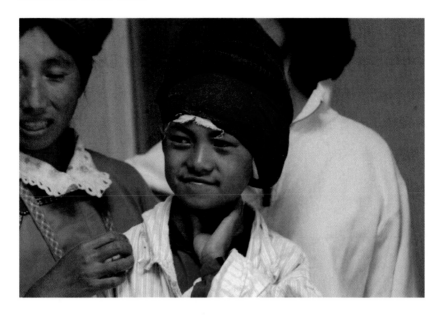

The audiologist wrapped up. The moment for Li Bing's first-time hearing words had arrived, as we were ready to turn on all electrodes together for the first time. I think of it like a symphony warming up—each instrument making a single noise until, finally, the beauty and awe-inspiring sounds come together as one. Normally a family member receives the honor of the first words. His father spoke. "Li Bing, can you hear me?" he asked.

"Yes, Papa, I can hear you," the boy replied. That was it. That's all his father said. The look on the faces of this family of three as they looked first at one another and then to us was indescribably precious. In that brief moment, something valuable that was lost was regained.

Some would judge their relationship as one bereft of love based on such minimal communication. But they would be wrong. From those few words the translator conveyed, I gauged that a mighty love lay beneath them. The meaning those words truly transferred, the message behind those punctual, concise syllables uttered in that small room, can't be fully expressed. The weight can only be felt, not explained. As with so many other parents of patients in so many other stories in this book, that man's face couldn't be described. I would have a better chance of getting an Eskimo to understand what humidity feels like, or a Thai fisherman what snow feels like, than I would expressing this joy—the joy that makes some leap up and down, run outside, and exclaim the reason for their jubilee—I saw in his face.

There was a relief too in both parents. After their son spoke, they stood a little less rigid, a little less like soldiers on guard. After four days of waiting, after four days and four nights of watching their boy and watching us work and incise and insert and tinker with technology they had never seen, unsure whether it would function, whether Li Bing would hear again, or whether they would be faced with a crushing disappointment. Now they had their boy back. We were separated in language, but as parents, joined in the mutual spirit of love and concern for offspring.

After some well-shed tears of joy, attendants brought in refreshments. But before I could partake, our translator took me aside and said Li Bing's father wanted a private word. I happily obliged, and the three of us stepped outside.

"I know why you came here," he said.

"Yes," I replied, rather flippantly. "I came here to place a cochlear implant in your son."

"No," he said. "That's what you did here. I know why you came here." He now had my complete attention. I realized he could be about to address my always present question, wondering if we had chosen the correct site for this trip.

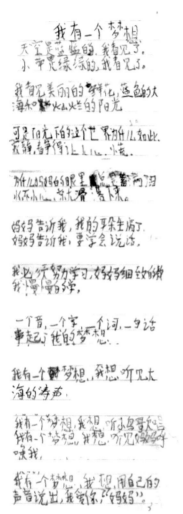

I have a Dream
The sky is blue, I see it
The grass is green, I see it

I see the beautiful flowers, blue
ocean and bright sunshine

But why this world feels so lonely
and so silent

Why Mama's eyes are full of tears
tear drops are running down her face

Mama told me, my ears are sick
Mama told me I need to learn to speak

I need to learn speech diligently
I slowly learn to speak under Mama's
caring guidance

From one sound, one word,
one phrase and one sentence,
They string my dreams together

I have a dream, I want to hear
the sound of the ocean wave

I have a dream, I want to hear bird chirping
I have a dream, I want to hear my Mama calls
my name

I have a dream, I want to use my own voice
to say " I love you, Mama"

"When my son became deaf, I was so sorry for him, and I was so hurt at the misfortune he had suffered," he explained. "I expressed my hurt to my friends, and they helped me. You see, for one full year before we heard of your trip, my friends and I gathered together before the sun rose each day before we went to the fields. When we came together, we prayed to Jesus that he would heal my son's deafness. Jesus brought you here."

The faith that Chinese farmer from a tiny mountain village exhibited is an exemplar to me. It proves that God moves via unseen channels. That father's vulnerability in gathering friends in a plea to God for help—help with a type of technology he had no idea even existed—is a testament to his true strength as a man.

That simple, desperate prayer brought a physician and medical staff and 20+ others all the way from Silicon Valley America—the most prosperous, wealth-generating region of the world in the history of the world—to a remote grouping of huts in a rural region tucked deep in the heart of one of the world's most formidable communist heavyweights.

It taught me something about my Maker's heart. You simply cannot go through an experience like that and not know you have been gifted to enter a holy event. God sees value in His people, and not only hears them but answers their requests. He sees people suffering and, in Li Bing's case, sent alleviation.

Our Maker, in His great sovereignty, marshaled resources, transportation, talent, technology, and political favor to send those of us willing to serve over a long bridge—impassible by man's effort alone. At the end of it lay the target of God's affection—people, specifically a little Chinese boy named Li Bing. Until that moment, it had not been crystal clear we were going where we were supposed to go—now it was.

12

I Don't Even Want to Know

2008

TO DATE, OUR ENDEAVORS have been fairly successful. Each program we have worked with continues treating patients with cochlear implants—miraculous devices that impart hearing. As of this writing, we have placed 75 or so implants worldwide in nine different countries on LTHF week-long trips. Now over 4,000 devices have been implanted—that's 4,000 people who won't be limited by deafness, who will be free to work and live in a world of unmuted beauty, unfettered by a disability that keeps so many from hearing the incredible sounds God created. So far, each program has continued growing for the good of their local patients.

The first step to get an LTHF program functioning efficiently and independently requires a few components. The first, and probably most important, is a healthy dose of interfacing with local surgeons. We seek to train them to be autonomously functioning professionals and to support them until they get there.

Email has also been a God-send, bridging the distance made so readily apparent by a geological gap, and allows me to stay in constant connection with surgeons who'd be otherwise nearly unreachable. Frequently, I receive queries that include scans, clinical history, and examination, etc. questioning how to handle certain situations.

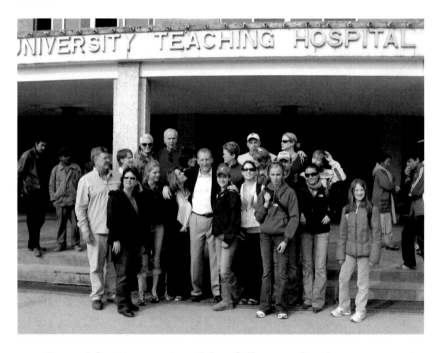

Stateside, I'm assisted by fellows who have committed to one or two years of additional training—on top of the nine they have already completed—as a final step, a final refinement of their skill in ear surgery. In contrast, the internationals I work with have far less experience. Experience varies from each individual, but it's often years less than the fellows I work within the United States—hence their far greater need for guidance down the line. Since our time at each location is sometimes severely limited, it's more of an intense crash course than anything else.

Also, some things simply can't be taught in a classroom or textbook. Outside of basic, technical surgeon skills—those can be sharpened and developed through training—we watch carefully for qualities found in a surgeon's disposition; some call it instinct–the ability to make judgments and decisions with confidence regarding patients while under pressure. They are a surgeon's pearls, sixth senses that require the same patience the former demands. Medical school or not, if a surgeon can't make tough decisions when the well-being of patients is at stake, their effectiveness is severely hampered.

For greenhorn local surgeons, their first real operation is an understandably nerve-wracking one. Aside from the difficulty and challenge of implanting a device into a cochlea, a complex organ buried deep in the inner ear, the fact that every cut, every incision, every decision they make could damage a sensitive area and organs virtually impossible to repair weighs heavily on them.

So before they begin a procedure, I show them a series of slides, a roadmap that systematically breaks down and gives a detailed glimpse of each stage of the operation. For some, it's new information. For others, it's a repeat. Regardless, it's a step I do my best not to let them skip. In surgery, inexperience is treacherous; the procedure a surgeon is least familiar with is most likely to go wrong. Sometimes we examine human cadavers in place of slides if they're available. For the surgeons, this is far more enriching than slides, as it gives them a tangible, realistic specimen most like that they'll be working with.

We don't often use the full body of a deceased person, but only the head, as that's all our operations necessitate. Some may interpret using a human body for some strange, scientific end as a grotesque or disrespectful gesture. It is indeed quite brutish, maybe even Frankenstein-esque, but as physicians seeking to heal people, it's our obligation to prepare ourselves as best as possible within ethical boundaries.

To safely perform an operation as delicate and risky as a cochlear implant, we must know what we're working with. The human body is a wondrous creation fully inspired and crafted by God, a supercomputer no human could ever reproduce. It's an incredible privilege to study it, learn how it works, and, hopefully, discover ways to better heal it.

We don't take our work lightly. I personally do my best to respect the deceased individual whose body provides vital information and education. We, as surgeons, owe an incredible debt to those who donate their bodies to medical teams like ours to improve care for those yet to be treated.

Unfortunately, sometimes necessity forces medical professionals in poorer countries to make do with less than the ideal. Some don't have the opportunity to examine the specimen of a human body. Others lack the expensive, highly advanced equipment we use in numerous procedures.

I often face this reality in my trips abroad, which causes deep introspection. How do those born in a nation lacking the abundant opportunities to learn and flourish cope? What if our roles were reversed? How different would my medical abilities look without the luxuries I currently enjoy as a physician? Could I overcome such challenges?

God, I think, keeps me humbled with these musings, which force me to look at the world through a lens of gratitude, one untainted by national identity, and made all the clearer by my citizenship to a higher kingdom—the kingdom of God.

A decade ago, we were in Nepal and had four implants scheduled for our team of Nepalese surgeons. Our team of 20 or so people included an OR nurse, an audiologist (who instructed local audiologists how to program the cochlear implants), two members of the board of directors of LTHF and their families, and several other donors who wanted to observe the amazing experiences firsthand. We were all eager to see the Himalayas and were disappointed when the cloudy cover of winter obscured the view as we landed in the capital.

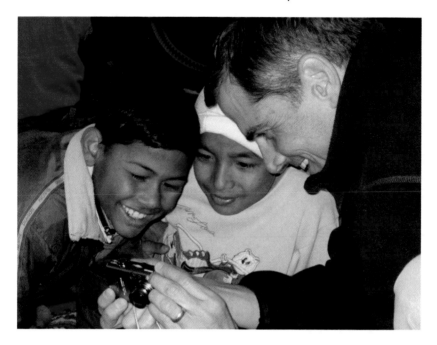

On the first day, we met the families and explained what was to come in surgery, programming, care of these new devices, and how best to habilitate children who would soon hear for the first time.

Per usual, we set some time aside one night before Monday surgery to run some pre-surgery classroom sessions with surgeons and physicians in the area. The room bustled with faces, young and old, from regions near and far. We started with slides, and I lectured and fielded some excellent and pointed questions pertaining to technique from both the trainees and members of the audience—a positive indicator they were engaged and learning something. I was glad the implants would be performed by individuals with sharp aptitudes for adapting and learning quickly, and I was humbled to work with

surgeons who performed procedures with whatever supplies and tools were available.

After questions and answers, I moved to an OR we set
up to perform simulated surgery on a cadaver head. I had
my surgical instruments arrayed as I always do before operations—a sort of ritual—an operating microscope hooked
up to a larger screen, one big enough to give the entire
class a detailed picture.

This equipment must be in the country, and I like to
use the equipment my trainees will be using to make sure
the quality is adequate for them to achieve success. My
OR nurse had traveled with us (a testament to her dedication, as she is petrified of airline travel). Her job was to
care for and deliver the other tools I needed to perform
this procedure—drills, scalpels, hundreds of tiny and var-
ied small tools we use to get into the human body to
leave the modern miracle of the implant while minimally
disrupting critical-to-life tissues. This, too, has a huge
amount of education and learning value to the surgeons,
as they have never seen many of our tools. It sometimes
makes for an interesting time in customs—and this country
had been no different—but that's another story!

I was armed and ready with everything I needed, save
the cadaver. Time passed, and, after a while, I inquired
when they would be bringing it in (a cadaver doesn't exactly choose when it shows up). I wasn't impatient or worried, just curious about the amount of time it was taking.

The clock ticked on, and still, no cadaver, so I asked
again. "Almost there, almost there," they retorted. "Just a
few more minutes."

I asked myself why it was taking so much time to
wheel in a corpse. I have dealt with stubborn patients, but
I was sure this individual was not resisting a visit in any
way; maybe the gurneys in Nepal were just slow.

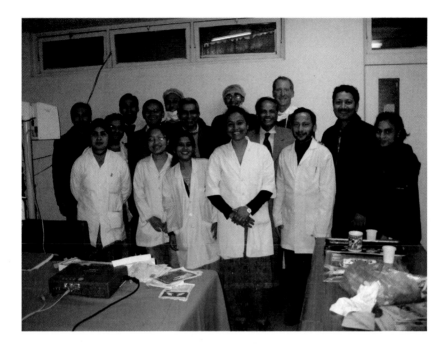

I turned to my audience, using what would have otherwise been idle waiting as a teaching moment. "It has been said practice makes perfect," I told them. "But it's more accurate to say perfect practice makes perfect." They nodded in agreement, some even writing out the phrase on paper. I continued, articulating the importance of practicing on a real, three-dimensional model—that such an opportunity gave not only surgeons but their patients something to be truly thankful for. The more acquainted surgeons could grow with the feel, pressures, sound, and other tangible elements of a surgery, the better the chances of success, I explained.

Fifteen minutes later, the staff and our special guest arrived. "Finally," I thought, relieved our long-awaited "patient" had come, momentarily oblivious to the unusually long time it had taken. Most surgeons are the hands-on, "put me in the game, coach" type, and I'm no exception. I shifted my chair, took a final look at the attendees, focused my attention on the task ahead, and got set to dive in.

As I grabbed the head, however, I was struck, by an innate feeling that not all was in order. A moment later, the veil of ignorance fell, and the realization rushed in blaring sirens of alarm that rang loud and clear—this head was still warm. In previous demonstrations, the cadaver had always been cold. I had handled plenty and never noticed until now.

Before that incident in Nepal, I had never handled a human head that wasn't cold. But here was a human head that, despite its appearance, was radically different from any other specimen I had handled. A river of questions came flooding in—How long had this cadaver been, well, a cadaver? Was it simply stored somewhere warm, or was it only moments ago a living and breathing patient? Had they passed consciously or unconsciously, painfully or painlessly? I didn't have answers and, in retrospect, thankfully none were provided. To this day, I'm unsure if the Nepalese present could see the surprise on my face. Sitting there in my chair—shocked at the strange and disturbing nature of this particular specimen—with attendees eagerly waiting to scrupulously examine the delicate procedure, I simply pushed on and told myself, "I don't want to know. I don't even want to know."

13

Spoon Intubation

2009

TWENTY-SEVEN. That's how many of us made the trek to Kunming, China—an ancient city in China known for its cherry trees, lake concourse, and women with large and beautiful eyes. The journey had been arduous, but we had yet to begin our work. While the medical staff and my staff would be doing cochlear implants, the other members of our party would visit orphanages, offering help however they could.

The first morning, I awoke to an inky black twilight at 4 a.m. Travel has a way of completely thrashing any shred of a sleep schedule. Besides, I was restless with the same sort of anticipation that woke my kids somewhere around the same time on Christmas morning, excited to jump into the day ahead and all it holds. No one else had woken yet. I don't get many moments of quiet and solitude in my line of work, especially while traveling.

With a corner of the clock reserved, I prayed for oversight, guidance, and direction as I contemplated the day ahead. I felt a slight nervousness, par for this course, and I could almost taste it in my prayers. My team and I would be the first to perform a cochlear implant in the region of

China, stirring excitement with both locals and the media. We'd already pre-screened five recipients and selected a surgeon and team of physicians to accompany us for training. Our goal was to leave this functioning team in place to carry on the work with our advice and support from afar.

The previous night, I had given a translated lecture on cochlear implants to a group of medical students, physicians, and local luminaries. Watching the early morning darkness slowly fade, I recalled mental pictures I had snapped of them–their curiosity, their eagerness, all of it held back with a professional seriousness. Later that day, I spotted stories of the event plastered on the front page of the newspaper.

As the sun maintained its unceasing course past the morning horizon, the team awoke, gradually filtering into the breakfast area of our hotel. Each helped lug down surgical instrumentation, programming computers, and a monitor I used for the implant surgeries; all of it had survived a pass through customs and the journey. Spirits were high. Team members spoke and ate quickly, lively and excited to start the work.

Most of them had traveled around the world to perform medical work in a country they had never stepped foot in; western China, in particular, has been mostly untouched by modern technological development as we knew it. It's a rural area surrounding a small city by Chinese standards, only 6.5 million. The native farmers, their quaint villages, the food, all of it, the vibrancy of novel communities, makes a stark impression on visitors, particularly those who enjoy the luxuries of a first-world country.

Around 6:00 a.m., the team gathered in the hotel lobby. We were scheduled to start surgeries at 8 a.m. at the hospital; our transport would arrive a half-hour before that. While we waited, my surgical nurse prepped our equipment, ensuring it had remained sterile.

After drumming up some conversation with a few of the younger team members, I stepped away. I checked my watch and glanced around the room, counting heads and visually checking our containers of equipment.

At that moment, I felt a still but strong urge that I should go to the hospital early. It wasn't a voice, or a vision, or even a word. I didn't hear or see anything. I only felt a nudging, a quiet, soft feeling deep in my gut that was a clear communication. I obeyed, almost without thought. The feeling, subtle as it was, was strong, firm, certain. The decision nearly seemed instinctual.

Appointing another team member as coordinating lead for the trek to the facility, I said I would meet everyone in the OR. I then left alone and walked the half a dozen blocks to the hospital. The city streets, now lit with the sharp brightness of a newly arisen sun, were crowded with hordes of commuters bustling about. The streets were crowded but different from those of an American city. The thousands of local residents were quiet. Bikes, not cars, provided transportation second only to the numbers on foot Fleets of them zoomed in hushed herds about the urban blocks, flowing like moving water around those, such as myself, who'd opted to use legs over wheels.

As a six foot, three-inch-high white man crowned with red hair, I was an obvious outlier, a blatant deviation from the locals, whose hair was a beautiful glossy black, and who generally measured between five and five-and-a-half feet in stature.

A few minutes into my journey, I arrived. After finding the OR, I greeted the first patient's family we had met the night before and dressed before proceeding into the OR. By then, the hospital staff was readying themselves to put this family's daughter under with anesthesia. After a brief greeting, I started checking my equipment, leaving the anesthesia staff to their duties. In one corner of the room sat a fellow native of the Silicon Valley—a pulse oximeter—a monitor that beeps and provides readings of a patient's vitals, particularly their blood-oxygen saturation levels. This technology was part of China's equipment and had provided a marked reduction in the risk of anesthesia since its commercialization and manufacturing by two American companies in the early 1980s.

This OR staple functions by passing a specific wavelength of light through a patient's fingernail, over which a small, wired clamp has been placed. The signal displays the absorption patterns of oxygen in the blood via a wavelength on the monitor manifesting as a number that corresponds to the percentage of oxygen the blood is carrying compared to its maximum capacity. For ease of use, that number is expressed as a beep with every heartbeat—a sound that currently pervades every OR anywhere. The higher the percent of saturation (a good thing), the higher the pitch of the beep. Conversely, the lower the percent of saturation (we get concerned with anything below 90 and move to action with anything approaching 70), the lower the tone of the beep. Chances are, you have heard its trademark beeping noise in some Hollywood portrayal of a hospital.

Two women were at the far end of the room attending to the girl. Per protocol, they administered medications that induced unconsciousness and complete, physical relaxation. During this pre-phase of surgery, patients require breathing assistance when they go completely unconscious, as they cease breathing on their own. An anesthesiologist inserts a tube into their mouth with an L-shaped device called a laryngoscope, holding the patient's tongue up in one hand and the endotracheal tube in the other. They push it through the vocal cords and down into the passageway leading to the lungs, called the trachea. On the other end of the tube, a machine is attached, which pumps air in and out of the lungs—artificial breathing, if you will.

If the person inserting the tube mistakes the esophagus—which leads to the stomach and is parallel and just next to the breathing passage to the lungs—for the trachea and places the tube there, a patient won't get the air they need into the lungs. If left in this state, they effectively suffocate without even knowing it. Fortunately, the pulse ox monitors provide an early warning, in this case.

I was still looking over my instruments when I noticed the pitch drop of each successive heartbeat, a sound surgeons dread. It was slight at first, but no less disturbing. I had heard that beeping noise tens of thousands of times, if not millions, of times. It was small but, to me, rang like a siren on a fire hydrant. In one swift motion, I set my equipment aside, stood, and strode to the anesthesiologist, covering the width of the room in a few quick steps.

Though I would normally be able to diagnose and handle this sort of situation with relative calm and coolness, the language barrier became painfully obvious, and the direness of the whole thing rocketed upward. Although the dialogue of doctors trying to place the endotracheal was lost on me, their speech was tense, verging on anxious, growing in speed and aggressiveness. The tube, it seemed, hadn't been placed correctly.

My attempts to learn more were met with the same fruitfulness of an endeavor to carry sand in a basketball net. After 30 seconds of unsuccessful attempts at verbal communication, the whole operation that started with a rhythmic mundanity that marked so many others had turned into a full-on emergency. The pulse oximeter pitch droned menacingly to a lower and lower pitch as the oxygen in the blood was being depleted by the patient's living cells, reaching life-threatening levels.

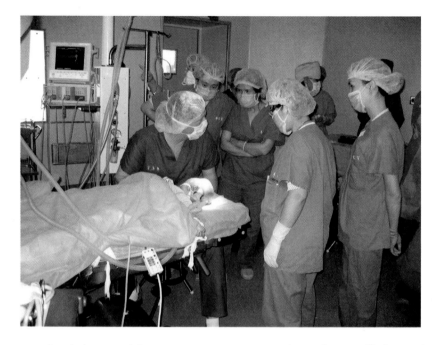

And then, without a pause or warning, the staff darted out of the room. For a few seconds I waited, simply stunned, casting out lines of optimistic hope; maybe they had gone to fetch help; perhaps there was a piece of equipment they had realized was missing. A few moments passed, seconds, probably, but they felt like hours.

My waiting and hoping proved as futile as my tries at speaking to my now absent staff. I was left alone in the OR with the girl, whose skin had turned a blueish violet, deepening in hue by the moment.

A newspaper headline flashed across my mind— "American Doctor Kills Chinese Child!" I was looking disaster in the face—things could turn ugly for my team and me if this girl died. We could be barred from helping other children, and our credibility would be destroyed; hopes for future trips could be dashed if she didn't leave that OR alive. And still, most importantly, her life was now pushing closer and closer toward a deadly edge from which I had to pull her away.

I quickly moved over to the head of the table. I procured an Ambu bag—a product of 1950s medical science created just for this sort of situation—and used it to squeeze air into the endotracheal tube. I squeezed again and again. Each time, I could hear an empty blowing sound. A few more tries and I figured out air was going through her esophagus. I looked for a mask to ventilate her without a tube in her trachea—something we would always have on standby in our ORs—but found nothing. A chill ran up my back. If the tube was down there, then it wasn't getting oxygen to her lungs and, thus, her blood. If this kept up, her heart would go into an abnormal rhythm, which would soon kill her.

I looked desperately for a laryngoscope, scraping desperately past equipment, tubes, machinery, papers, anything that may have masked the tool I now so dearly needed. Time ticked. I looked again. By now, her face was turning a dark purple and, still, no laryngoscope. I had come so far, over so many miles, and, despite my fears, I felt a charge of aggressive determination; fear took a back seat and my urge to save, to heal, to do what I was born to do, jumped in the driver's seat. So the laryngoscope was missing? Fine. It wouldn't stop me. Find another way and quickly! I had to find alternative measures.

While I hastily scanned the room for anything I could substitute for the missing instrument, I remembered seeing a small spoon on the counter in the room next to the OR. I ran in, found it in its original location, and grabbed it, dashing back into the OR and bending the utensil into an L-shape. After quickly adjusting the overhead lights, I pushed over and behind her tongue and pulled the endotracheal tube out of the esophagus.

Inserting the bent spoon under her tongue, I inserted the tube into her trachea where it was meant to be in the first place. After reattaching the Ambu bag, I squeezed it.

For a few moments—as tense as piano wire—the pulse ox monitor's steady beep droned on at the same, flat pitch I initially so dreaded. It takes 10-15 seconds for oxygen to enter the lungs, be absorbed by the blood starving for it, return to the heart, and then be pumped out to the finger where the pulse oximeter sensor was located. But then, as quietly and subtly as the first change, I heard the pitch rise ever so slightly and then return steadily to 100%.

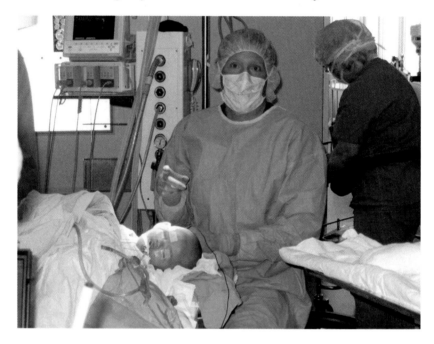

Minutes later, a crowd of Chinese hospital workers crashed into the room, all of them talking in quick, worried speech. To their utter shock, they found me sitting by the head of the girl's bed, smiling and gesturing with my hands as if to say, "Why don't you take over now?" I didn't want to even think of the stories that could have been told if this precious child had not been snatched from the jaws of disaster that morning.

As I left the room, I looked down at my watch. 7:30. My team was only just now leaving the hotel. If I hadn't gotten there early, hadn't followed that nudge, I'm not sure what would have happened to that girl—well, actually, I think I do know what would have happened. Sitting in the prep room, waiting for my team to arrive, I breathed a relieved sigh, happy that the girl not only would survive but that I had heard and listened. My heart froze at how easy it would have been to ignore the prompting I heard early that morning in the hotel. Oh, and I kept the spoon.

14

Colby

2010

COLBY TURNED SEVEN like millions of other children in America. She was raised in a regular household, by a loving father and mother. She attended school and kept good grades. For some time, her life differed little from the average American fourth grader, but shortly after her birthday, Colby was assaulted by an ailment. She started vomiting, went lame, lost hearing in one ear, and lost control of half her face.

A friend and former trainee, who'd opened his own practice in our area, examined her. An MRI revealed an apricot-sized lesion of her skull base adjacent to the area where the spine joints join the brain.

Her parents took her to the five best and brightest surgeons they could find across the United States, including my clinic. Each examined her, and each reached similar conclusions—unknown. Simply put, they couldn't diagnose it because none had ever witnessed anything like it, especially in this age group.

The situation called for a tissue diagnosis. This entailed surgically removing a piece from the lesion, freezing it while the operation is ongoing, placing a razor-thin sliver of it on a glass slide, staining it with special stains, and placing it under a microscope for examination to determine the type of tumor tissue. Using the instrument, an experienced neuro-pathologist—they specialize in tissue from, in, and around the nervous system and brain—can usually gauge the nature of the lesion. It could be a tumor that grew in that spot or one that metastasized from somewhere else in her body.

Colby's family asked me to do her surgery. It needed to be soon, as this was progressing and wasting time was not in her best interest. Since I had no time on my surgical schedule for several months, we needed a solution. I discussed it with my family, and we felt it was a good idea to take the first portion of our vacation to go to war for this young girl. Normally, I'm swamped with multiple patients, but Colby came on a day my office was normally closed; she'd be my sole focus.

I hate to watch children suffer and personally anticipated the chance to battle on her behalf whatever disease or ailment or infection caused her suffering. She wasn't just a person who needed healing, and I happened to have the skills to help; I wanted to champion her. I would want someone to do the same for my own children if I were unable to. The confidence families and patients place in me is perhaps the greatest compliment I ever receive.

The focus and singleness of purpose of a group of men and women dedicating their time and talents to a child—one single, overwhelmingly important goal—is such a beautiful thing to me it's hard to relay. At 6 a.m. sharp, my team of nine highly trained and specialized surgeons and staff readied themselves and the necessary equipment. A pediatric neurosurgeon arrived, who'd come at Colby's parents' request in case something went wrong with her brain.

We needed specialized pediatric anesthesia techniques and postoperative care not available in the adult hospital, so the operation took place in an adjacent pediatric hospital. The hospital is wonderful, but unfamiliar environments are less than ideal when performing work as delicate and dangerous as this would prove.

Even tiny differences in the way equipment works can mean large differences in outcome. Diana, my hardworking, dedicated nurse, transported my usual tools to the pediatric hospital. That's a lot of equipment, including my microscope, which is valued over many homes and weighs more than some automobiles. Uneasy about working at an unfamiliar location with unfamiliar facilities, tools, and instruments, including even the lights and anesthesia machines in the OR, Diana's labors—and the tools she brought that I was accustomed to using—provided me a needed cushion of comfort, confidence, and success.

For an hour, I watched every detail of the team's preparation. Weeks before the surgery, they had labored, straining over every detail, over the logistics of every stage, every moment of the procedure. Now was time for *esse quam videri*—which means "to be rather than to seem to be." It's one of my favorite phrases. There was no hiding now, only the harsh reality of one outcome that we were solely responsible for as a team. Oh my goodness, do I love that kind of task!

I found Colby with her mother and father in the pre-surgery holding area. I recognized the feelings shown on their faces. They were the same ones I felt when I cradled my 30-month-old daughter Caitlin in the emergency room, praying to God to spare her life. If you're a parent, you have probably felt those same concerns at some point. Colby's mom was especially anxious; the girl was her only child, the baby she and her husband tried for years to have.

I did something I have found comforts every parent whose children I have treated—I touched them as I looked into their eyes, laying my hands on their own, relaying my confidence that my team would work with all the resources, ability, and heart we had. I reassured them that we'd attempt to do the surgery perfectly, or as best we could, and, most importantly, that all of us cared deeply.

I remember the eyes of the parents. It's my addiction actually—the same eyes before and after the work is done. When someone asks me what the hardest thing to give up will be when the time comes, I answer, "The OR waiting room." I usually have to explain that what I mean is the joy I see in those who have entrusted their precious loved one to us when they hear "all is well."

My gesture eased them some. They handed over their girl, and, about a half hour later, Colby left the conscious world as she went under anesthesia.

With Colby asleep, I inserted monitoring electrodes near her face, mouth, throat, and neck to keep watch on the nerves the tumor had wrapped around. The staff took care of the bladder catheter, an arterial line, and an intravenous line, and administered antibiotics, all while calibrating the herd of monitors and machines that provided us live readings of her vitals. After shaving off a patch of hair behind her ear where I would enter her skull, I taped off the area where we'd be making an incision. To reduce the bleeding, we injected Colby's skin with anesthetic agents and epinephrine.

We finished prepping her, and I left the room, leaving Diana to place the sterile drapes on the patient to wall off the incision and wound from bacteria and other germs in the non-sterile parts of the OR. Other surgeons were shocked I let Diana handle this. In general, few doctors would ever entrust a nurse with a task like this or even think about doing so. I think for many of them, it's a matter of pride to allow a nurse, someone ranking below them, to do their work.

I understand most of those doctors have studied a lot longer than the average nurse, but that doesn't validate the former's treatment of the latter. Nurses are invaluable, possessing as much heart and fight as some of the best surgeons. As Diana proceeded, some of the team cast glances of shock in my direction. I paid them no mind. They were good people, not prideful; most just didn't have the privilege of working so closely with a single nurse like I did (and still do). Since I was the only surgeon in the hospital to employ my own nurse and we had worked together for over a decade now, Diana knew how to complete this step perfectly. Ironically, I had removed a similar tumor from Diana's husband years before, which led to us working together.

By now, my attention was cast through the glass separating me from Colby, who lay amid hundreds of thousands of dollars' worth of medical equipment, all crammed into that 25'x25' space for her sake.

Before an operation starts, we meticulously wash our hands at the scrub sink just before we "gown and glove" to begin the procedure. After the hubbub of preparation, going to sleep, patient positioning, monitor placement, etc., it is a somber moment of calm.

My mind drifted to a Christmas song from my childhood.

> I played my drum for Him, pa rum pa pum pum
> I played my best for Him, pa rum pa pum pum…

We each have our own grown-up version of "The Little Drummer Boy," I suppose, and this was mine. It may seem silly, but it helped me stay calm and concentrate. More importantly, it's a reminder of the why behind what I do—to serve him with my skills and training—at the forefront. I asked myself, "Would you do this any differently if it was Jesus himself under those drapes?" That is an intense question and one I have suggested to others in any line of work to find out if they are doing their best. Colby deserved that special of an effort, and I was going to give it to her.

Diana's work finished, we entered the OR. Save for the AC that hummed above, it was quiet.

I wasn't the only one who tasted the weight of the situation. Normally, an OR is a noisy place, and aside from the machines, surgeons crack jokes, chat with each other, sometimes in silliness, sometimes crudely, using the same sort of workplace jargon people in other professions do. This time, though, their voices were hushed, somber, spared for only the most necessary phrases. Their body language told the same story; they were tense, faces serious, bodies rigid, movements stiff. I think some were nervous about the outcome. After all, no amount of surgical expertise can fix many of the things we are afflicted with on this earth. Although such a blanket of quiet can help productivity, anxiety can clout a surgeon's ability to think and act decisively. It's like trying to run a 5K through streets flooded with molasses.

As I donned a gown and gloves, I realized only Diana and I had performed this procedure before. Only my two fellows (apprentice surgeons training to learn these skills) observed in similar operations before.

The silence was pervasive, damming up higher and higher every passing moment. The situation felt like it teetered on a slippery edge, sloping down toward panic, danger, emergency for many of the staff in the room—something too scary to imagine. What if we killed this child trying to help her?

Perhaps worse, what if she was left with permanent damage that significantly altered her life? In reality, each of those could happen. Thinking of them at this moment, however, was completely fruitless and can be paralyzing. Turning to the fellows, I broke the silence and asked them if they were ready. They nodded. I calmly and confidently said, "Yes, we're ready." It helped; that simple action changed the mood in the room, shifting the tension off our shoulders.

The tumor was buried deep—about three inches under the patch of skin behind the ear I had shaved earlier. Cutting a tiny slit parallel to the back of her ear, I incised delicately, exposing her skull. The work was done through the microscope as I sat to the patient's side, her head turned away.

After stemming the bleeding from the scalp tissues, a specialized drill was placed within the field. After 30 minutes or so of drilling at 60,000 rpm, I reached the location where the jugular vein, ear canal, facial nerve, and brain lining intersect. A suction tube clasped in my left hand and the drill in my right, I washed away bone chips as I delved further, all the while watching through a microscope. It was like managing a construction site full of powerful and dangerous tools while watching from a hot-air balloon with a telescope.

Nearing the tumor, I noticed the bone adjacent to it had eroded and thinned to a skimpy one or two millimeters in thickness. Where healthy tissue once walled up, now little more than paper separated the motorized bone shredder in my hand from vital brain structures bathed in a gin-clear liquid surrounding all brain structures, called cerebrospinal fluid. Peering into it, I could see the brain covered by a latticework of veins and arteries that pulsed with every beat of her heart.

No time for unsteady hands—or an earthquake for that matter (they're somewhat common in southern California). I held my breath intermittently to reduce movement in my own body. If any one of those structures snagged on my drill's blade, they would wrap around it, and the torque of the drill would tear them away. It would kill Colby. I felt like I was descending a well, a well with walls I couldn't touch in a space suit with binoculars strapped over my eyes.

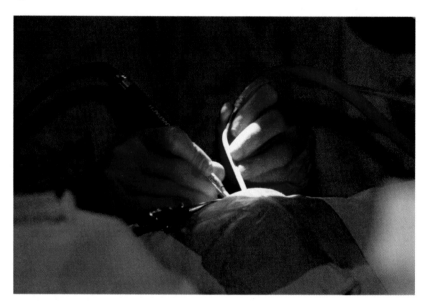

What felt like a long time of bone removal finally yielded sight of the dura, a tissue that separated me from the tumor and is the natural dividing tissue between the bone of the skull base and the brain cavity. The tumor was just on the other side of the dura, and I had to re-move all the bone on this side to allow a full view of it for safe removal. Otherwise, I would be working through a smaller keyhole than I already was working through.

Trading my drill for a pair of small, sharp neurosurgi-cal scissors, I snipped a path through the dura. As soon as I did, my stomach dropped— something felt wrong in the tissue. I had cut through the dura many times before and it didn't feel like this. Could malignant tissue be laced in the structure of the dura? What's more, the tumor itself was not easily separated from the dura—a rarity. In 1,000 separate cases, I had never seen anything so strange. I couldn't diagnose the problem—not right away, at least. Our neuropathologist would do that when I provided a piece of tissue for staining and examination under high-powered microscopes.

Further examination of the tumor showed even more extension and damage. Like a gumdrop exposed to heat, it was soft and sticky, adherent, the consistency more solid than that of firm scrambled eggs. However, this gumdrop was alive and, on its lower side, had bonded with an artery vital to Colby's survival. In an expanding, blob-like process, the now deadly lump of tissue had also stuck to nerves that controlled the girl's swallowing, her voice box, and trapezius muscle. The tumor was alive, and the damage it was doing clearly characterized it as insidious. The top of the damnable thing had also pushed up into another vital vein, draining the upper portions of the brain.

After some careful and demanding dissection freeing fractions of a millimeter at a time, I completely separated the tumor from the dura. It gave us better access to the tumor. I could now see around it 360 degrees if I moved my microscope on its robotic control arms to peer around the corners of the remaining skull base. As I had observed before, the vocal and facial nerves were enveloped, badly.

I had warned her family of the possibility that in order to fully remove the tumor we'd need to cut the facial nerve—a necessary evil. We'd repair them with a nerve graft sewn in place for the missing segment, yes, but Colby would lose control of her face for some time, and the final result would never be normal—just a partial amount of disordered movement.

After seeing the nerves so ensnared in the tumor, I began thinking we'd actually go through with it—we'd have to or risk leaving a viable tumor. Then I thought of the years of healing and therapy Colby would need to speak again if we had to cut the nerves that controlled her voice. Her quality of life would be hampered. It would be tough on the girl, growing up that way.

We wouldn't give up yet. My resolve to preserve the nerves strengthened. I brought the neuropathologist in the room to look over the problem with me. It never hurts to have an expert see the tumor in its native state, not just in a specimen dish, especially when you're dealing with someone's brain and nerves.

With him watching through my microscope, I snipped off pea-sized pieces of the dura and the tumor—his analysis of the samples would dictate our next move. Before he tested them, he informed us of the two most probable, realistic, options he foresaw: if the tissue proved malignant—dangerous or toxic—we'd have to remove it, including the nerves it had attached to; if benign, it was harmless, and we could save the nerves and only remove parts of the tumor.

He marched off to conduct testing. No one talked for a while as we prepared to close the wound where we'd bored and cut. I could tell the team was nervous. Even Diana, the nurse whose nerves seemed to be made of iron, wore a concerned expression. They knew the consequences of cutting those nerves; they knew the quality of life the girl would have if we did so.

Thirty minutes or so were required to analyze the tumor appropriately. As I mentioned before, the tissues had to be stained with specialized reagents and sliced microns thin to be placed on slides and evaluated under specialized microscopes in a room away from the sanctum of our OR. It was a long time to wait surrounded by the beep-beep-beep of Colby's heart as the monitor tracings displayed and moved.

Our tissue evaluated, the neuropathologist reentered with a verdict, commanding everyone's attention but directing his comments to me. I was still sitting in my surgical chair with my gown, gloves, and mask on, hands crossed, hoping for good news. The tissue was benign, a harmless schwannoma tumor! If mood was temperature, the room got a whole lot warmer as the good news swept away the concern that had been brooding among us. We had hope. I called out Diana's name. Before I got any further, she interrupted me.

"Yep, it's going to be ok. Let's go get it," she said, articulating our thoughts.

The staff dimmed the overhead lights as I pointed the microscope, the only device emitting illumination at that point besides the pale blue-green glow of the anesthesia monitors. The bright, white beam of light was streaming toward the gaping wound under Colby's ear, exposing the now-vulnerable undersurface of her brain. I felt like all the times I had suffered, pushed myself, and sacrificed to work as a physician, culminated in moments like these. Yet somehow, they paled in comparison to such a task, one that my Creator had now entrusted to me. When I am in situations like these, I never wish I had done less to be ready.

Face your fears—take them head on, by the horns, starting with the one that scares you most. That's what I teach my fellows when they work in an OR. If something makes them nervous, I push them to deal with that first. Since it has proven the safest pattern of action in my own experience, I forced myself to do the same with Colby.

Pulling all of my concentration into a microscopic point, I moved in to free one of the two veins most at risk—cutting it would inflict the worst damage, leaving Colby with a massive stroke, never to recover. Its thinness made it difficult to get at with my micro-instrumentation—too much applied pressure, and I'd penetrate the two-tenths-of-a-millimeter-thick wall of the vessel with disastrous consequences.

The work had to be done intermittently, like a pearl diver who uses no oxygen tank and apparatus and must constantly return to the surface for air. Colby's breathing machine naturally increased the pressure around her brain with every needed breath and flooded the cavity I worked in with the clear fluid naturally surrounding the brain called cerebrospinal fluid (CSF). It can't be removed as the brain must be only partially exposed while it floats in this fluid. I was in and out, and then in and out again, and again, and again with my metal instruments, working delicately and methodically, nicking off a tiny segment of the tissue sticking to the vessel each time.

Fearful doesn't describe how I felt. More like overwhelmingly, incredibly focused. Knowing even the slightest interference could bring my operation to a bloody halt, I warned the team against touching any of the machines Colby was attached to. I even admonished them to cease any sudden movements, even coughing. My whole world of consciousness felt packed into that tiny incision. Perhaps one day we will have surgical instrumentation that extends the human capability to remove tumors like this, but on this day, the physical act was at the limits of human ability under the best and most pristine conditions—conditions my team had achieved.

In those difficult moments, those complex and dangerous operations, I'm perhaps weirdly most aware of God's joy. I think it's the mark He has put on me; it's what He has purposed my hands to do. Regardless of my years of school and training, my own wavering human ability, He works in and through me. It feels like He's smiling at me, watching calmly and peacefully. I haven't seen it with my own eyes as you see a beautiful sunrise or sunset, but I know it as sure as any truth.

After some more gentle handling, the vein was freed. I insulated it from the tissue I had just cut it from by wrapping it in a special type of shredded Teflon, not unlike a tiny cotton ball.

I moved on to the second vessel—an artery that was the only blood supply to the part of Colby's brain that provided her breathing and blood pressure. It was a bigger and more robust structure and, thus, easier to distinguish from the delicate vein now protected under a barrier of Teflon, but it moved and pulsed with every palpitation of Colby's heart. "Life is in the blood," I thought. It's not just literal but a symbolic truth for believers.

Detaching that artery took even greater coordination than freeing the vein. Without that $600k microscope, I couldn't have done it. But once again, thanks to careful cutting and coordination, I had freed it. After that came a few nerves to the vocal cords, the shoulder musculature. They don't pulse and were probably the easiest to free. Millimeter by millimeter, I swept them off the tumor, ever so gently breaking the delicate connections that held them to the intrusive invader.

The tumor had emerged from the lining of the balance and hearing nerves and infiltrated them, creating a tapered, hourglass shape. Choked of life, the balance and hearing nerves were dead. They were dysfunctional and had gone, as they contained tumor tissue throughout their lengths. Nearly completely free of arteries, nerves, and vein, Colby's unwelcomed guest, the tumor, and the facial nerve it pinched and choked—keeping Colby from controlling her face for the last several weeks—remained the last obstacle. The nerve was a 1.5 mm-wide strand of tissue softer than overcooked pasta—its consistency resembled cooked egg whites more than anything—that would tear at the tiniest tug, killing it and forcing us to graft a new one in place for Colby. Again, caution almost didn't seem enough.

With one hand, I stabilized the tumor against the sling of the artery I previously freed—the only vessel in the vicinity with the tension to withstand the pressure I applied—which served as a cable. Cutting the tumor from the ear side of Colby's head toward the brain, I found the nerve, whiter than the pinkish interior of the tumor. I swapped the scalpel set for a special instrument I designed specifically for cutting a vein or artery, or even a nerve, free from both sides at once—a sort of double scalpel. Carefully, with the greatest of my own ability, I cut away the tumor around it. The nerve free, I finished off the remnants of the intruder, pulled it out, and handed it to Diana. Even with a surgical mask covering her mouth, her smile showed. All she could say was, "Yep."

Only the dura remained. I wasn't totally sure if it needed to come out, but there was something wrong with how it had grown, and I didn't want to take any risks. The neuropathologist advised against it, but I knew if something was wrong with the dura, Colby would pay for it later. Plus, as a surgeon—and more importantly, as a parent—I couldn't in good conscience tell her parents we did our best if we didn't take it out. Now was our best chance; we had a good shot, and we'd already had success. I decided it was the only way forward.

I thought back to the question I had pondered while I scrubbed my hands—what would I do if Jesus Himself were in this room, on this table? In Matthew 25:40, Jesus said helping "the least of these," was helping Him. If I were operating on Him, I had to leave no option off the table; no procedure would be too great, too difficult, too challenging. I would do everything I knew to treat Him to the best of my ability. Therefore, doing my best—helping, doing something right, healing—is the approach I choose to take, regardless of the patient.

The dura is a tough and fibrous tissue about 1-1.5 mm thick that is densely adherent to the inner surface of the skull and skull base. It is the boundary or sac that contains the cerebrospinal fluid the brain floats in during life.

In this case, the benign tumor had grown into the dura—a fact I had first noted when I cut through the dura and it felt different from healthy dura. Painstakingly, I incised the dura widely around the affected area and removed it from the bone with sharp dissection, preserving the structures that left the brain to proceed to the remainder of the body—a delicate process.

Satisfied, I irrigated the wound, removed the Teflon I had left around one of the remaining nerves and any other non-viable tissues in the cavity, and halted the bleeding with bipolar cautery, a form of cauterizing that doesn't risk damaging delicate nerves and brain tissue. Fat from the abdomen was harvested and packed into the bony defect cavity.

After the surgery, it lived and grew, and scarred into the opening. In that way, I dammed up the CSF leak by sealing off the eustachian tube and the middle ear. Otherwise, the dura removal could lead to a leakage of CSF into the back of the nose. Even worse, bacteria could go the other way and enter the brain cavity, producing life-threatening meningitis. In our final step, we sutured the skin and underlying tissue in several layers in a watertight fashion, lay special tapes on the skin over that, and then placed a firm dressing on top of it all. Except for my three trays of tools—Diana didn't pack them up right away in case an emergency forced us to reopen the wound—the nerve-monitoring equipment and microscope were shuttled off.

The anesthesia lasted for about 15 minutes before Colby woke. Heart rate and brain function were stable on the anesthesia monitors still connected to her. Colby regained her own breath, and the breathing tube was removed, although we still watched her closely until the staff transported her to a recovery room.

Colby's harried parents had waited for 2.5 hours without hearing a word about their daughter. They sat, holding each other close in the waiting room, bracing, I think, for the worst sort of news. Some people say being watched activates some a sixth sense. I can attest. I felt the eyes of those parents zeroing in on me before I spotted them, I, coming to deliver much-anticipated news and, they, eager for word on their daughter.

There's a strange intensity to being watched when you carry something of weight, something significant. It's an intensity only parents who love their children–to the extent they would sacrifice themselves for their child– possess. I sensed they were uneasy, concerned, anxious, even breathless. And that's when I told them the news about the tumor, about the successful extraction, and, most importantly, that their girl would be all right and that I felt we had God-given success today. It didn't register immediately with either parent–too much goodness to take in, I guess. I repeated myself, and her mother grasped my message.

"Oh, OH, OOOHHHHHHH," she said. And then, "You mean you are … done? There's no bad news? I was waiting for bad news."

She leaped to her feet and then off them; her exuberance would have put a cheerleader to shame. Completely undone by the good tidings, Colby's parents collapsed in one another's arms, weeping and, from my perspective, not needing to say another thing. Into that hospital they had come, faces full of fear, carrying a girl physically tormented. Later that day, they left the anxiety of the waiting room with a whole and healed daughter, their faces illuminated by joy.

As I said earlier, the day wasn't a busy one besides this surgery. Rather than rushing off to another assignment, another situation, another emergency, I walked slowly, deliberately, from the wing of the hospital housing the OR to the intensive care unit (ICU), to the dressing room, and then to my car. I couldn't–still can't–thank God enough for the work He allows me to do. I never want to take what I do for granted.

God's heart, I believe, must be massive. He sees the suffering of millions and cares for us lowly creatures down here on this little planet. And here am I, just a man, who can only take on one hurting person at a time; it's all I can bear emotionally. This inadequacy is even greater juxtaposed with His power and might, His perfect love and healing power. I pray He comes soon. It would be nice to get worked out of my job.

Prompted by the verse below, and just like Colby's parents, I too shed tears of joy while in church the next day. I imagined a mother riddled with fatigue but bearing a tender smile, watching her young daughter sleeping in the ICU while monitors gently beeped, keeping watch on her recovery.

> Then I saw a new heaven and a new earth, for the first heaven and the first earth had passed away, and there was no longer any sea. I saw the Holy City, the new Jerusalem, coming down out of heaven from God, prepared as a bride beautifully dressed for her husband. And I heard a loud voice from the throne saying, "Now the dwelling of God is with men, and he will live with them. They will be his people, and God himself will be with them and be their God. He will wipe every tear from their eyes. There will be no more death or mourning or crying or pain, for the old order of things has passed away." He who was seated on the throne said, "I am making everything new!" (Rev. 21:1-5)

15

The Gift of a (Near) Death by Sandwich

2014

AFTER CONTRACTING CHOLERA during a trip to Peru, I lingered between a small hospital room and eternity. Death lingered close–the closest it's ever come to taking me, it seemed. In the end, I walked away alive, with a gift I could not have otherwise received.

We first visited Peru in 2004. During the trip, we performed 10 cochlear implants (an astounding amount of work) on children all roughly ranging in age from two to four years old. Ten years later, we returned and did five or six more. On this second trip, we were able to see the children we treated during our first trip. The implants we gave them then enabled them to speak, so seeing them older and communicating through speech was immensely rewarding.

During this second trip, I also had to perform an unexpected implant. The staff, my wife, and I had been getting ready to visit Machu Picchu–an old Incan castle of sorts, now in ruins. It's a tourist hotspot, and we wanted to bring our staff along.

On these sorts of trips, people sometimes become overwhelmed with the experience, so we make a point to give ourselves something to take their mind off their work.

Our plan was to fly out from Lima and spend a day or two enjoying the area and visiting the ruins. I was looking forward to the trip, excited to see the old relics history had left behind for us to enjoy.

However, shortly before we departed, a mother reached out to us, urgently pleading on behalf of her child who desperately needed an implant. Needless to say, I forwent Machu Picchu.

Just before we started the surgery, one of the staff members asked whether I was hungry. It was around lunchtime, and I was indeed, but as the experience of international travel dictated, I remained cautious and asked what the meal consisted of. He informed me it was simply a sandwich he'd prepared at home, and my stomach grew louder than my inner voice of common sense. I gave in, assuming it was relatively safe, and enjoyed it just before I began the surgery. For a while, I was fine and brushed off any concerns I still had about the meal.

Time passed, and, for the most part, I forgot about the sandwich. Unbeknown to me, this was the calm before the storm.

Near the end of the surgery, I noticed my GI tract was getting active. Too active.

I finished the surgery and started heading back to the hotel room. It was a downhill slide from this point. Afterward, I was told my health deteriorated so rapidly, it started showing in my physical appearance. I was shown a video someone took of my van trip back to the hotel as evidence. Watching the video now, I can honestly say that I looked like death warmed up. I got back to the hotel and, assuming it was simply GI disturbance, temporarily assured myself I would be all right. "I have been here, done this before," I told myself. I couldn't have been more wrong.

When I finally got to my room, things escalated quickly. Explosively quick–literally, both ways–to a point at which I was as astounded as I was concerned. It was bad and getting worse–and fast. Pretty soon, I was losing fluid at an unnaturally fast rate, and it steadily grew worse. I was being pummeled, mercilessly.

A couple of hours into the misery, my wife returned from dinner.

"You don't look good at all," she said. "You okay?"

She's never seen me miss a day of work, so you can imagine her concern when I told her I needed to get to an emergency room.

My anxiety was starting to mount. I was severely ill, and being this sick anywhere, not to mention a foreign country, had me on edge.

My body continued expelling fluid. By now, the loss was so great it was affecting my blood pressure, which was so low that just sitting up would make me pass out. I even started raising my feet because it was the only way to get enough blood into my brain and keep me–semi-alert. And even in implementing this maneuver, which seemed to take a superhuman effort, I was still weak and constantly faded in and out of consciousness.

Meanwhile, my fluids kept flowing–just as fast too. Articulating the process is difficult. I can only say it felt like there was a garden hose on full blast plugged into my intestines–that's the best way I can put the feeling into words. It was so voluminous and intense that, after only an hour, the fluid coming out of me had no color. All I could think was, "Wow, this is intense."

After a quick call to a surgeon friend (we needed advice on which hospital to go) and a brief cab ride, we arrived. My wife, who doesn't work in the medical field, was unsure how best to aid me in my half-conscious state.

Fortunately, one of the patrons who spoke Spanish came with us. She'd already been to Machu Picchu and had decided to stay with us. She lit a fire under the hospital staff, spurring them into the proper course of action, (In retrospect, the fierce urgency she conveyed probably saved my life) and soon I received IV fluid, a vital component for keeping blood pressure steady.

It's a scary feeling for physicians in an emergency room to realize they're the ones who need help, unsure if the local staff know how urgent the situation is. As a surgeon, I was accustomed to helping people, not needing help. But there in that emergency room, I experienced a role reversal.

Only four to five hours earlier, I was operating and performing an extremely delicate procedure under a microscope, in a controlled, environment with high-tech equipment. And now, hours later, I had become a helpless patient, unknowingly etching my way steadily toward the verge of leaving the planet for good. I was no longer the captain of the ship, but a helpless crew member, hoping to survive the storm that raged inside my body. The reversal illuminated how transient and fragile life can be.

I eventually got out of the emergency room after four liters of IV fluid, checked into the hospital, and told my wife to go back to the hotel so she could rest. "I'll be fine," I told her. "Things are good."

"Okay, you know what, I'm feeling much better now," I told myself, trying to bolster my morale. "This will turn around."

Again, I completely underestimated the severity of my illness and continued losing fluid at an alarming rate. However, the evening nursing staff lacked experience and didn't believe me when I told them I needed more IV fluid in broken Spanish (which only exacerbated our misunderstandings). It was a fight, a battle of pulling teeth with pliers that didn't work. Back and forth, back and forth.

"Necesito más. I need more fluid," I told them again and again. Again and again, my requests were blown out of the sky with a rapid burst of, "No, no, no, no, no, señor, no."

During the–12 hours that followed, I only received about 22 liters of fluid. I'm a pretty big guy. My whole circulating blood volume is somewhere around six to seven liters. Those 22 liters were far from enough, so holding onto consciousness remained a constant struggle. Between the times they had me plugged into IV fluid, my blood pressure dropped so low that my brain would begin to malfunction. Somewhere around 2:00 a.m., during this wrestling match with mental fogginess and doubtful nurses, the reality of my situation became startlingly apparent–this night, I realized, could well be my last; I might not survive.

I couldn't contact anybody. Save for the beeper on my bed used for calling nurses–I'm sure they grew sick of hearing it as the night wound on–I was left bereft of any way to communicate with those outside the hospital.

Every 10 to 20 minutes, my IV bag of insufficient fluid would run dry, and every 10 to 20 minutes I paged them to come change it out.

Compounding the difficulty of staying awake and alert was the battle I had to fight just to use a toilet. Since the toilet wasn't near the bed, I had to get out of bed and walk to it. Sounds easy, and normally would be, but half the time I rose to start the 10-foot journey (that at the time it felt like ten miles,) I passed out almost immediately–a testament to how dehydrated I was and the lowness of my blood pressure.

The hours ticked on. Somewhere in the darkness of that night, around 3:00 a.m. or 4:00 a.m., the realization that my end could be near, that death may be just a few more empty IV bags away, became clear–crystal clear. "Dude, this may be your last day on the planet," my brain told me. That triggered a floodgate of observations and questions. I remembered the surgery I did earlier and the sandwich I ate. "Not what you were thinking when you came to Peru for implant surgeries." Ironic. Cruelly ironic.

But then, different thoughts fluttered in: "It's a gift, in some ways, to face your mortality and to stand, really have to stand and look at how fragile life—especially your own—really is," I observed.

I thought of my family too. "Will they be all right when I go?" More questions followed: "What is your life made of and did it count? How did you do? What grade would you give yourself?"

These thoughts worked their way around my brain for some time. I held them there, pondered them, and even tried to answer them. All my worries regarding my purpose, to happiness, to satisfaction and self-worth, they all came bubbling forth that night of physical suffering and pain. Somewhere deep in the night, I reached a place where I was comfortable if this was my time to leave.

Eventually, the darkness passed. I had survived the night.

The next morning, a surgeon we had worked with at another hospital, and his wife—a pediatrician who deals with many infectious diseases in patients from developing nations similar to Peru—came to visit. She took no more than two steps into my hospital room when there on the spot, she diagnosed me with cholera. She could discern the sickness simply from the odor the infection produced. Now I remembered a long-ago lecture on the subject and the words, "Improperly treated cholera carries a 50% mortality."

The lightbulb had been switched on; I had received improper treatment because no one, including me, knew the cause of my ailment. They had been using the wrong antibiotic to treat me. That's like trying to put out a gas fire with water.

Soon after, we changed my antibiotics to the correct ones, and, in a short period, the downhill course turned around. I had recovered.

It had all happened so fast; funny how life sometimes works that way. That last cochlear implant surgery was on a Friday afternoon. Friday night, I checked into the hospital. Saturday, I got the proper antibiotics, and Saturday evening, I was discharged. Sunday morning, I was on a plane to California, and Monday, I operated on a patient there.

Looking back is like recalling a nightmare. But I think I learned something there, lying on that bed, dying in some Peruvian hospital where the staff either didn't understand or didn't believe me.

But I think I took home a gift from that harrowing ordeal. I had to ask myself, "If I leave today, did I leave anything undone? What should I have done with my life?" I suppose it took almost losing my life to fully evaluate its worth and to live in a way that I'm ready to leave when that day comes. That realization is a gift, and a heavy one at that, but as heavy as it is precious. It's one I'll treasure forever.

Oh, and next time someone offers me a sandwich that was possibly made under less than ideal circumstances, I'll probably turn them down. I'm sticking to Powerbar for a little while now.

16

A Prayer

2017

DINNER HAD GONE COLD. It'd been hours since I'd excused myself from our host's table, feeling nauseous. Since then, there'd been no letup to a vicious onslaught of vomiting; had to have been something in the food—not from dinner, that is, but from before—a foodborne illness I'd acquired sometime before dinner. I was miserable, low on fluids, and feeling worn thin from throwing up and, eventually, dry heaving.

It was all happening while we were on one of our trips performing cochlear implants; this time, in Costa Rica.

All I wanted was rest, but dawn came, and the coming surgeries loomed ahead. Granted, I'd only be performing two, but still, each would require immense focus and effort—both traits that are normally strengthened through sleep, of which I had little to none.

However, I'd been trained to battle through exhaustion. My sickness would have to take back burner to the more pressing issue of surgery.

There was one patient I was especially eager to get to. His name was Jose David, and we had a small window—

one day—to operate on him. "Calling in sick" was not going to be an option today.

Sometime late in the morning, or early in the afternoon, I stood at the head of Jose David's stretcher. Some staff and I formed a semicircle around him, praying for safety and a smooth operation as we do before surgeries. That day, our standard practice took on new meaning.

I took the moment to glance at the others standing nearby, something I normally refrain from during these prayers. Unlike myself, their heads were bowed, their eyes shut in earnest piety.

To my surprise, someone else was there with his eyes open: my three-year-old deaf patient. He was looking about at those standing adjacent his stretcher, his eyes showing some sort of earnest curiosity, innocent, and fearless.

Then, his face moved quickly to look up beyond those around his bed. His face showed recognition, joy, excitement, and peace as he looked past me and into the air. He reached up like a child who wanted to be picked up and held. I couldn't see anything he was seeing, but he clearly "saw" a being that comforted him—something that was powerful, loving, reassuring and beyond our usual realm. His reaction and the words of prayer gave me a sense of being surrounded by a larger power and purpose that cared deeply for this boy's welfare and life. At that moment, I grasped my position as a participant in a much larger tapestry that goes well beyond an operating room in a small country in Central America. At that moment, a photographer caught the scene in the image you see here.

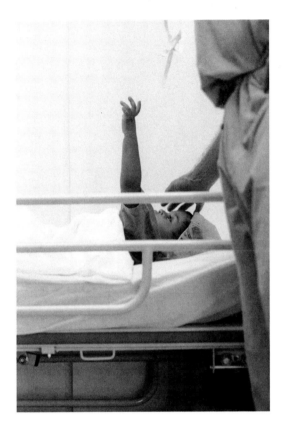

That moment was truly an anomaly, unique and unlike any other I'd experienced during a prayer before surgery. I knew then that things would be all right, that God was looking out for this boy, myself, and all the other staff working to heal his ears. That simple action brought so much hope, so much encouragement.

Before the prayer ended, his hands dropped back to his side. Only he and I (and the photographer) had shared that precious "vision" while others kept their heads bowed and eyes closed for the beauty of earnest prayer.

In that moment, I wasn't so tired. For all I knew, the food poisoning was a distant, dull memory. The surgery went along perfectly, and days later, Jose David heard sounds for the first time.

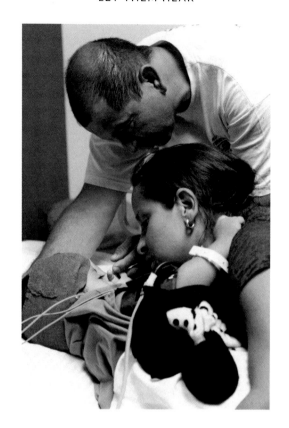

About Joseph B. Roberson, Jr., M.D.

AT THE START OF HIS CAREER, Dr. Joseph B. Roberson, Jr., M.D. served as the Director of Otology-Neurotology of the Skull Base Surgery Program at Stanford University. During his 10 years at the university, he focused on hearing-related brain tumors and cochlear implants as well as a small number of patients with an ear malformation present at birth called Congenital Aural Atresia & Microtia (CAAM). Since 2004, he has served as Chief Executive of the California Ear Institute Medical Group and its many related medical entities.

In the 1990s, there was still a great deal of room for improvement in the treatment of CAAM, and the need for a center of excellence for the condition. Dr. Roberson began to focus on CAAM and established the International Center for Atresia & Microtia Repair and Global Hearing to respond to this need and to focus on this condition with a goal of improving results.

In 2002, Dr. Roberson and his wife started The Let Them Hear Foundation, a non-profit Christian organization that helps treat deafness in children and adults. Since then, the foundation has provided assistance to set up multiple cochlear implant programs around the world, including training surgeons and staff. More than 100 Surgeons have been trained through this program while Dr. Roberson has performed more than 100 cochlear implants in international venues personally. Due to the programs LTHF initiated, more than 5,000 deaf children in countries around the world have received the gift of hearing through a cochlear implant.

At this time, Dr. Roberson's main focus is the surgical care of children and adults with CAAM. He has treated over 3,000 patients from over 55 counties around the world. He still cares for many patients with a wide variety of ear- and skull-related disorders.

A Personal Note from Dr. Roberson

No one wakes up every day for their entire life ready and excited to go to work. By nature, work can be—and frequently is—full of mundane drudgery that seems boring and hard to endure. In some cases, however, work brings our existence into focus and causes us to ask the greater questions "why am I here?" and "who am I here for?"

As a father, I have marveled in the processes my own children experience as they choose how and where to spend their work lives. I can see their gifts and personalities so clearly having seen them grow and mature. Watching them 'become' is one of the more enjoyable processes in which I have ever been engaged. In addition, I watch their friends in their early adult years. I am mesmerized at the process as it unfolds so differently for so many different people. I delight in getting them around our dinner table outside on a warm California night as other family members and I pepper them with questions. Sometimes they love the topic, and other times it releases quite an inner storm of emotions and fears and uncertainties.

At different points in my life journey, I have interacted with men from many different professions as they consider their work and how they came to do what they do. In many cases, the path was chosen for them by family or a cultural norm. In some cases, a prior family member has made such a successful business of one type or another that it naturally draws a man into it. There are as many paths to a life's calling as there are humans on the planet.

What I have learned in observing these very private revelations is it is relatively rare to align one's gifts and natural abilities with his/her life purpose. Sometimes that is just the way life is. We all need to eat and have shelter and work provides these things. In many phases of life that's ok as a means to survival.

I realized in a weekend away with 100+ men in my early 40's that the alignment of work and calling has occurred for me. I can't say that I can take all the credit by trying to achieve that myself. It has grown to be something I am deeply thankful for. I grasp it is a rare and tremendous blessing.

What I want to encourage you to do is to seek to align your purpose/s and your talent/s. The reason I think that is a good idea is because of all the men and women I have seen closely in this subject area, the ones that are the most satisfied and fulfilled with their work are those who have achieved this alignment. Most people who achieve the alignment I speak of have many different iterations of it over their lifetime in differing jobs and phases of their lives.

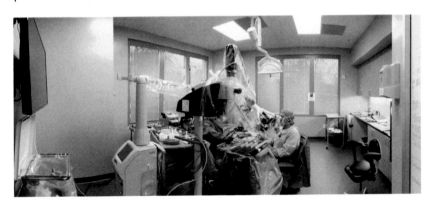

Many different online tests, books, and professional service organizations exist to help you determine your 'giftings'—those things you are especially good at doing—such as your interests, personality type, values, interpersonal relations style to name a few. I am sure there are those in your life who would share their thoughts on the subject, too, especially if they have watched you move from childhood on to later life stages. Ask them! Search for what you are made of and what brings you joy with engagement.

When you find it, next search for what you were made to do with those abilities. You may have to search for a while to be sure you have it right. It took me over a decade to be relatively sure.

I believe there is a Maker—as you now know reading this book—who designed you for a purpose from before you took a breath. I know life doesn't seem like that sometimes, but the more I go along, the stronger this belief has become in my heart and mind. If you know your Maker, ask Him and then listen very, very carefully and patiently for answers on the subject. They will come. If you don't know your Creator and want to, I suggest and even challenge you to read the book of the Gospel of John in the New Testament in the Bible. (There are other books of John in the Bible, but you want the first one in the sequence.) Read it with an open heart to see if your Maker wants to open a relationship with you. I would be willing to bet one of my fingers that I know the answer to that question!

Lastly, the stories in this book are highlights and don't think for a minute my life and work are all giggles and sunshine. I love the stories you have read here to be sure. Many of them describe situations where I can see in my mind's eye my Maker smiling as I work. I have just as many where I was frustrated beyond words, tired, bored, and frankly sick of work and out of patience. My point is this—nothing good comes without a lot of effort preparing and making yourself ready. Stories like these are few and far between, and that's what makes them valuable to me. It is unrealistic to think you'll walk into a situation with all the skills and abilities to achieve marvelous things overnight. You can do great things, but sometimes it takes years. If you think about the totality of my life, it took decades for some of them to emerge. Many times, you will do great things and nobody but you (and your Maker) can see them. Still, you will know when they come.

Keep at it with fierce tenacity and be singularly focused on your target when it comes into view. There will be times—maybe years from now like it was for me—when you are called on to bring what you have and to serve people when no one else could have. That is beyond satisfying, and in my opinion, that is the best we can feel about work.

In the meantime, and between mountain peak and valley experiences like you've seen here, keep pressing on. May the Maker of Heaven and Earth bless your efforts and encourage you along the trail.

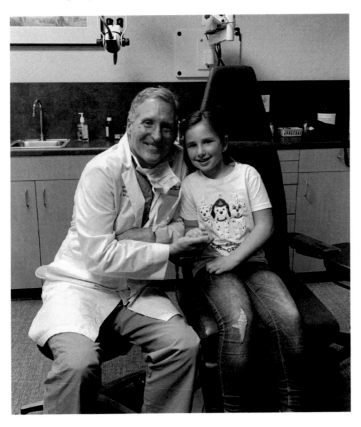